SHOCK

AVERY

a member of Penguin Group (USA) Inc.

New York

SHOCK

The Healing Power of Electroconvulsive Therapy

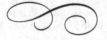

KITTY DUKAKIS

and

LARRY TYE

Published by the Penguin Group

Penguin Group (USA) Inc., 375 Hudson Street, New York, New York 10014, USA • Penguin Group
(Canada), 90 Eglinton Avenue East, Suite 700, Toronto, Ontario M4P 2Y3, Canada (a division of
Pearson Penguin Canada Inc.) • Penguin Books Ltd, 80 Strand, London WC2R 0RL, England •
Penguin Ireland, 25 St Stephen's Green, Dublin 2, Ireland (a division of Penguin Books Ltd) • Penguin
Group (Australia), 250 Camberwell Road, Camberwell, Victoria 3124, Australia (a division of Pearson
Australia Group Pty Ltd) • Penguin Books India Pvt Ltd, 11 Community Centre, Panchsheel Park,
New Delhi–110 017, India • Penguin Group (NZ), 67 Apollo Drive, Rosedale, North Shore 0745,
Auckland, New Zealand (a division of Pearson New Zealand Ltd) • Penguin Books (South Africa)
(Pty) Ltd, 24 Sturdee Avenue, Rosebank, Johannesburg 2196, South Africa

Penguin Books Ltd, Registered Offices: 80 Strand, London WC2R 0RL, England

Most Avery books are available at special quantity discounts for bulk purchase for sales promotions, pre-
miums, fund-raising, and educational needs. Special books or book excerpts also can be created to fit specific needs. For details, write Penguin Group (USA) Inc. Special Markets, 375 Hudson Street, New York,
New York 10014.

The Library of Congress catalogued the hardcover as follows:

Dukakis, Kitty.
Shock : the healing power of electroconvulsive therapy / Kitty Dukakis and Larry Tye.
p.   cm.
Includes bibliographical references and index.
ISBN-13: 978-1-58333-265-8; ISBN-10: 1-58333-265-0
1. Electroconvulsive therapy.   I. Tye, Larry.   II. Title.
RC485.D85   2006   2006022506
616.89'122—dc22

(paperback edition) ISBN-13: 978-1-58333-283-2; ISBN-10: 1-58333-283-9

Printed in the United States of America
9 10 8

Book design by Meighan Cavanaugh

CONTENTS

PREFACE

There is no treatment in psychiatry more frightening than electroconvulsive therapy. It works like this: Two electrodes are strapped to the patient's skull. The doctor presses a button that unleashes a burst of electricity powerful enough to set off an epileptic-like convulsion. The sheer strength of the seizure shocks the brain back into balance.

There also is no treatment in psychiatry more effective than ECT.

Ask any psychiatrist about it and he is likely to rave—provided no one is listening. Even more certain is that he will recommend ECT only as a last resort, if then, and will barely refer to it when training the next generation of psychiatrists.

Mention it to someone on the street and the first reaction is: "Shock treatment! They aren't still doing that, are they?" Often followed by, "My aunt Agnes had that a long time ago and it made her better."

How is it that a therapy nearly seventy years old still provokes such passionate and paradoxical responses? No remedy in medicine is more entangled in polemics than ECT. This book sifts through the controversy and unravels the contradictions. It separates scare from promise, real complications from lurid headlines. In the process, it offers practical guidance to prospective patients and their families on whether ECT can help them battle depression, bipolar disorder, and other disabling mental diseases. ECT stirs fears and hopes that intrigue everyone but mystify most. This text is an exercise in demystification.

It does that in two voices, one personal and narrative, the other dispassionate and explanatory. The narrative is Kitty Dukakis's experience with ECT, presented in every other chapter in the first person. Kitty knows about mental illness. For two decades she has suffered a depression that at times she has been able to outrun and at other times has marooned her in bed, unable to think of anything but the next mouthful of vodka. She also knows about the addictions that frequently accompany psychiatric sickness. Her unlucky romance with diet pills started at age nineteen and lasted twenty-six years. Her drinking began later and persisted nearly as long, although she has been sober for five years. Such dependencies and disease would be tormenting for anyone; for Kitty they were aggravated by her husband Michael's three terms as governor of Massachusetts, his 1988 run for the presidency, and her high-profile roles in all of them.

The explanatory chapters are mine. I am a former medical writer at the *Boston Globe*. I first heard Kitty's story when she and Michael told it to participants in the Boston-based training program that I run for health-care journalists. My fellow reporters and I sat transfixed by the tale of a treatment we were supposed to know about but did not, and by storytellers we thought we knew but had never heard speak so movingly. Their presentation had special resonance for me: A journalist friend had recently considered ECT when nothing else could lift him out of despair, but he was scared away by lingering images from Jack Nicholson's *One Flew Over the Cuckoo's Nest*. A favorite aunt had the procedure when I was a boy, and she was depressed and desperate.

Kitty and I began a negotiation en route to a collaboration. She had already shared her experience with friends of friends, along with total strangers, who had heard about her treatment and were searching for something to subdue their demons. Now she wanted my help bringing her story to a wider audience. I was reluctant to wade into the controversy but became mesmerized by a treatment that some condemn as torture and others lionize as life-saving. I said I would join in, on two conditions: that I could tell the broader story of ECT to fill out her individual angle, and that I would have the freedom to go anywhere the facts led me, for better and worse. She enthusiastically agreed.

Kitty's tale is more than just hers. It is the story she remembers, with recollections and reactions woven in from her children and husband, her sister and brother-in-law, and friends who, as always with a disease like depression, played roles in her illness and her recoveries. It is her struggle with alcohol and with diet pills, which both masked and exacerbated her despair. Her doctors contributed to this retelling, opening her hospital and therapy records to her and to me, adding perspective, and letting me observe as she got convulsive treatments over the course of more than a year.

My chapters probe ECT's history, its effects, and its prospects. They are based on interviews with leading ECT researchers and practitioners in the United States and overseas, some fifty in all. I talked to passionate critics, along with historians of medicine and others familiar with the procedure as it has evolved over the last half century. I visited ECT clinics across America. I pored through sixty books on electroshock and related procedures, and read about six hundred articles. Most important, I talked to people who had received ECT, more than a hundred of them, for illnesses ranging from depression to schizophrenia and with results that ranged from life-sustaining to personality-obliterating. Some were referred to me by their doctors. Others were sent by anti-ECT activists. Most came my way thanks to ads posted and e-mails sent by support groups like the National Alliance on Mental Illness and the Depression and Bipolar Support Alliance. While some asked not to be named, or to have us use just their first names, most spoke at length and for attribution.

My subjects were famous people, like Pulitzer Prize–winning author William Styron, and anonymous ones like Carrie DeLoach and Christine Elvidge. DeLoach, a thirty-two-year-old English teacher who lives in Spain, got ECT twice for deep depression and once for "a manic high like I'd never experienced." Each time the therapy restored her equilibrium, immediately and without a single complication. Elvidge opted for shock treatment after nearly a hundred medications failed to calm alternating bouts of mania and depression—and after she tried slitting her throat with a broken mayonnaise jar. ECT made her forget everything from her daughter's recent birthday party to whether she had a husband. "At the time I said I would never, ever want to have ECT again," says Elvidge, who is forty-one now and a mental health counselor in Illinois. "Later I saw how it had helped me get my life back. ECT is not easy . . . but I believe it's better than taking your own life."

Each person I interviewed had a story that was slightly different. Yet after hearing a hundred of them, patterns started to form. Their stories, together with Kitty's, are the grains of sand that reveal the broader landscape of electroconvulsive therapy.

Our book begins filling in that landscape in Chapter 2, which explores the dramatic yet subterranean comeback of ECT, then zeros in on what the treatment looks like today from the United States to the British Isles and Indian subcontinent. Chapter 4 looks back at electroshock's birth and growth from the late 1930s through the 1950s, when it was the psychiatric profession's treatment of choice. Chapter 6 documents how, after thirty years on the rise, it fell from grace and from most psychiatrists' tool bags. ECT rose again starting in the mid-1980s, and Chapter 8 looks at the scientific evidence of effectiveness that fueled the rebound. Not all of its effects are good, of course. Chapter 10 considers memory loss and other complications that have kept ECT under a cloud of controversy, along with ways to minimize that loss if not defuse the controversy. Chapter 12 reviews the mechanisms underlying electroshock, ones we know and others we guess at, and previews new brain-stimulation therapies.

Woven between are six chapters of Kitty's up-close experience with ECT. Her struggles and triumphs help bring alive my history, medicine, and science. We conclude with an epilogue of simple advice to would-be ECT recipients.

The picture of electroconvulsive therapy that emerges is of a treatment with enormous promise, especially for depression, the most omnipresent mental illness in the world. The U.S. surgeon general, the National Institutes of Health, and much of the psychiatric establishment agree that ECT presents a better prospect for relieving severe depression than even the best antidepressants or the sagest psychotherapist. It goes to work faster, which is essential for patients determined to kill themselves. It also is accessible to the elderly, pregnant women, the physically ill, and those who cannot tolerate psychotropic drugs. And it is not just for depression: ECT has an enviable success rate for a series of other debilitating mental conditions. All of which explains why a treatment that nearly vanished along with the lobotomy and insulin coma is here once more.

But the stigma has not gone away. That is partly because it was planted so effectively by books and movies like *Cuckoo's Nest* and *The Snake Pit,* and because any therapy that sends a current coursing through the brain is bound to be contentious. It also is because ECT can cause memories to melt away, in rare cases going back years and never coming back. Like chemotherapy, ECT is a toxic treatment for a crippling disease. Like any surgery requiring anesthesia, it carries risks. And like the electric paddles that cardiologists use to shock a fibrillating heart back into rhythm, ECT is not a cure but can offer relief and even remission.

No one is sure just how this is accomplished. Or, more precisely, researchers have endless theories and little consensus. The seizure could be key, or shutting off the process that produces seizures. It could center around the electricity, or the same biochemical reactions that make antidepressants work. Many patients prefer to think of ECT as somehow resetting the brain when it gets out of balance, the same way rebooting a balky computer sometimes fixes it.

These pages also steer readers through the claims and counterclaims surrounding ECT. We agree with doctors who say the treatment is dramatically more forgiving today than during its bone-breaking primordial days. We concur with critics who say ECT can and should be made even better by facing and redressing complications like memory loss. Yet we surely will draw the ire of true believers in both camps—proponents, for pointing out ECT's adverse effects; opponents, for strongly disagreeing with their call to ban a treatment that is helping millions worldwide. Our real audience is current and prospective patients. For them we compare electroshock to drugs, talk therapy, and other treatment alternatives, knowing the latter are less intrusive but less likely to provide fast, effective relief. We also calibrate ECT's potentially onerous side effects alongside the often more onerous prospect of bearing a debilitating disease like depression. ECT, it turns out, is neither a panacea nor a scourge, but a serious option for treating severe ailments.

Wading through such minefields, we realize that even our choice of a name for this procedure is sure to be explosive, the way it has always been. Its founders toyed with electroshake and electric shock, finally settling on electroshock. The press and public preferred the simpler and more evocative electric shock treatment, trimmed to shock treatment, then to shock. As part of its recent renaissance, promoters opted for the scientific-sounding electroconvulsive therapy. Even better, the laconic and vanilla ECT. Kitty and I made different decisions on what to call it in our respective chapters. She largely avoids the term "shock treatment," which she feels is inflammatory and not descriptive of a procedure that for her has been benign. I generally refer to it as shock treatment when that was the name it was known by, ECT when that came into wider use, and throughout as electroshock, the title Ugo Cerletti chose when he launched the therapy at his Rome clinic in 1938. We agreed to use shock in our title because that is the name by which most people recognize the treatment.

Whatever it is called, the story of ECT is, in the end, a lens into how psychiatry and medicine work in America. It is a world where analysts argue with psychopharmacologists, social workers split hairs with psychologists and psychiatrists, and consumers wrangle among themselves and with practitioners. Those fault lines run especially deep when it comes to the profession's most controversial treatment, electroconvulsive therapy. Nowhere is there a clearer demarcation of the debate between medical and therapeutic models of mental illness. It is counterintuitive to see a treatment as time consuming and tangled as ECT catch on in this era of Prozac and the quick fix. Most surprising of all, ECT is the only remedy in mainstream medicine that is expanding in use, receiving increased attention in research, and offering life-saving hope to tens of thousands of people, even as much of the public believes it is extinct.

One

AN ANNIVERSARY
TO REMEMBER

It is June 20, 2001, Michael's and my thirty-eighth wedding anniversary. It is also the end of my fourth month of depression, my crisis period.

I'm normally a person with enormous enthusiasm for and interest in the world. I am very involved with my three children. Every week I talk to John, Kara, and Andrea three to four times each. I normally call my dad, Harry Ellis Dickson, once or twice a day, and I go over to see him all the time, he lives so close. Michael and I have a very full social schedule. I'm involved with my sister, my friends, with life. I read two newspapers every day, the *Boston Globe* and the *New York Times*. I always have several books I'm reading. I am a social worker, and I try to help people who have problems, especially refugees. I always have three or four cases I am working on.

All that is just missing now. I look around at friends who are enjoying life and having fun. Fun and enjoyment are things I cannot even imagine. I don't speak to my kids on the phone, or to

my sister. Friends haven't heard from me in weeks. I do keep up
with Dad, but he calls me more than I do him. I just went to a
Boston Pops concert where he was conducting, but I was so totally uninterested and uninvolved that he expressed real concern
to Michael. The last two people I want worrying about me are
my father, who is too old and dear, and my husband, who has had
to worry for far too long. I drag myself to work and miss a lot of
it, staying home and doing a lot of sleeping. I don't want to go to
dinner parties; when I do, I make Michael take me home early. I
have run out of options and I don't want to drink.

These are the times when I am most vulnerable. Having a
drink is the only way of bringing me away from the horrendous
feelings I am having about myself, my lack of interest in anything.
It starts out as a glass or two of wine. It generally ends up with
vodka, as much as a pint. The alcohol is like an amnesiac—it takes
me away from the darkness. It certainly does not end the depression. I think I know how to control the drinking; John and the
girls think otherwise. They imagine getting a phone call in the
middle of the night, after I have done something horrible to myself. But when I can't see any light in a very dark tunnel, a drink
is the only thing I can think of to satisfy that overwhelming depression. Last night I was so afraid I was going to drink, I was so
shaky, that I told Dr. Welch he had to check me in here at Massachusetts General Hospital.

Today I am going to try the only thing left: electroconvulsive
therapy.

Corky Balzac, my friend and counselor, says she was the first to
talk to me about ECT. That was nearly five years ago, and she recalls my saying, "'Oh my God, no. Shock treatment!' You were
terrified by it." I have no recollection of that. What I do remember is being in the psych unit here at Mass. General for earlier
drinking bouts and depression. Dr. John Matthews asked whether,

when I begin sliding into depression and increase my antidepressants, it ever helps. I said "no." John knew my bouts of despair were getting worse, and was worried where I was heading. He asked Michael and me if we had heard of ECT. He began to describe it and asked whether we would be willing to look at a film about it. We watched two of them, and the videos were very positive, very specific. That was more than three years ago. Jerry Rosenbaum, my psychopharmacologist, was death on ECT at that time. He didn't think it was the right treatment for me. I was so convinced that my therapist, Roger Weiss, would be equally negative that I never gave him a chance to tell me what he thought.

Michael and I have our own reasons to be anxious. His older brother, Stelian Panos Dukakis, had it back in 1951, in what I think of as the treatment's Dark Ages but they tell me was its heyday. As Michael remembers, Stelian was a junior then at Bates, and doing really well academically. He also was the best two-miler in the state of Maine among college kids. He hadn't done a lot of dating but had feelings for a gal who was a senior at Lewiston High at the time, an attractive and fun person. He had no sign ever of any mental illness. He was on his way back to Bates from a student government conference at Brown just after this girl broke things off with him. He was crushed. He called Michael's folks and said he wasn't feeling well and was coming home. He just fell apart psychologically. Michael's dad, a doctor, sent him to see a psychiatrist. Shortly after, Stelian tossed a pile of sleeping pills in his mouth, attempting to end his life or at least blot things out. Michael was at home and remembers finding Stelian on his bed, unable to be roused. Michael's dad and Stelian's psychiatrist decided he had to be hospitalized, at a facility not far from Boston called Baldpate. They gave him ECT along with insulin coma treatments, which was a combination they often used at the time. Stelian was never really the same person. He put on weight, which was not like him, and there wasn't much affect there. There wasn't much communication. He had a zombielike look, which melted the heart of everyone who knew and loved him. Michael remembers Stelian saying he never wanted to go through shock treatment again.

My family, too, had experience with ECT, with a bit more upbeat outcome. Al Peters, my brother-in-law and close friend, got it more than forty years ago at Bournewood, a psychiatric hospital near where we live in Brookline. Al was drinking then, and had some paranoid feelings. It was a time when the earliest antipsychotic drugs were being unveiled and before they were widely available. ECT was the treatment of choice, the same way it had been a few years earlier with Stelian, and Al got six or eight sessions. "It erased everything fermenting in my mind. I couldn't remember anything three to four months prior to that," Al recalls, adding that the whole thing was stigmatizing enough that he never told anyone about it. Not until he heard I was considering it. At that point he talked to Michael, making clear that while ECT robbed him of months of memories, it also helped clear his psychosis. "I survived it," Al said, "and it helped me."

Both experiences were discomfiting in different ways. What happened to Stelian wounded Michael so deeply that it was a long time before he could talk about it, the more so since his brother was killed twenty-two years later by a hit-and-run driver. Al was glad he had had ECT but had suffered a loss of memory that would give anyone second thoughts about the procedure, at least the way it used to be done. Neither of us even knew they still were doing electroconvulsive therapy before John Matthews showed us the video and referred us to Dr. Charles Welch, the head of Mass. General's ECT program.

Charlie Welch is a very gentle soul. There are certain people in our lives who can really make a major difference and Charlie is one of them. We were so impressed with him when we first saw him three years ago that we had kept in the back of our heads what he told us about ECT: that it had an 80 percent success rate, but also probably would cause memory loss. We loved those odds, and liked his honesty about possible side effects. Charlie also said I was the perfect patient for ECT, given the severity and stubbornness of my symptoms and the fact that none of the drugs I had tried were getting me better. He looked me straight in the eye that day and said, "You're going to get better." He realized, as he told us later, that "you and Mike already had dived off the cliff of desperation and were just hoping for a soft landing." Charlie was precisely the man to wipe clean for us the tarnished slate of electric shock from the days when Stelian and Al had had it. We were ready to try it right then, but the day I was due to start I came out of my depression and Michael checked me out of the hospital. We had gone as far as explaining all about the treatment to my dad, and he felt anything that was going to help was worth whatever risk there was. We knew that if the time came again when we were desperate for a solution—some kind of positive action— we would go back to Charlie and ECT.

That time is now. Yesterday they admitted me to the hospital under the name Jane Dee, a pseudonym they use as a courtesy to protect my privacy after my twelve years as first lady of Massachusetts and Michael's long campaign for president in 1988. They gave me a very thorough physical to make sure my heart, lungs, and other organs could handle the procedure. Charlie also talked to Michael and me, as his medical notes reflect. "On interview today, she appears severely depressed, although she is very skilled at concealing it," Charlie wrote. "She has a gaunt facial expression, paucity of speech, speech latency, motor retardation, constriction of affect, and a hollow voice. Although I have seen her several times in the past, this is the most depressed I have seen her. . . . The interview clearly is an effort for her. After extensive discussion, she, her husband, and I agreed that a trial of ECT is indicated. We also agreed that doing the first treatment on an in-patient basis would be advisable, given her inability to care for self, and her self-destructive impulses regarding alcohol. It is our hope that after one treatment she will have experienced enough incremental relief that we can complete the rest of the series of ECT on an outpatient basis. She will be admitted this afternoon, and will commence ECT tomorrow morning."

I know I am ready, but lying here waiting for Dr. Welch, the image of *One Flew Over the Cuckoo's Nest* flashes through my mind. I remember them pulling Jack Nicholson down and at-taching him to the bed, then the convulsions where his body is just racked with shaking, violent spasms. And I remember how crazy he was afterward. He certainly didn't improve much, with violent headaches and all kinds of other very disturbing side ef-fects. It is not an image that reassures. I am a social being and I am concerned what people will think about what I am doing. Get-ting ECT makes you a full-fledged member of the mental health family. What am I doing?

My daydream is interrupted when Charlie walks in. He has come to get me. We walk side by side down the hall, quietly. Later I sometimes ride in a wheelchair, but not with Charlie, not this first time. We take the elevator down to the treatment room where they do all their ECT work. I'm nervous; Charlie can tell. Michael said good-bye last night and is teaching today. He's going to come in after my treatment to pick me up, assuming I am well enough to go home. This is not the way either of us planned to spend our anniversary.

Charlie and I reach the treatment area. Everything in the room, which they showed me before, looks new and different now. I look around. The ECT machine is over there, and looks surprisingly simple, like an old-fashioned stereo system. The rest of the room is a lot like the one I just left on the ward. No restraints, burly attendants, or any of the other props I remembered from the Nicholson movie. I am the first patient today. No one else is around. Charlie's ECT nurse greets us, with the anesthesiologist I met last night, and they tell me what's going to happen. It seems cold—I'm not sure if it is me or the room—so the nurse puts a warm blanket on me. They clip to my finger a device that measures the oxygen in my blood. They stick a bunch of electrical leads on my legs, arms, and over my heart, to make sure my heart is okay. They attach a blood pressure cuff to my arm, then insert an IV line into the other arm. The anesthesiologist comes over and says, "I'm going to give you a shot of Sodium Pentothal. You'll be asleep within seconds." I am lying down. He says to think of something bright and cheerful.

I think about flowers and a field of daisies. I think about Michael and our anniversary.

Two

IT'S BACK

*I*t was the medical madness of an earlier era, a remedy forever equated with thrashing limbs and obliterated memories. Now, at the same Harvard teaching hospital where Kitty Dukakis gets her treatment, twenty patients a week volunteer for shock therapy. All are tormented by depression too deep to defy or another disabling disease of the mind, and all, like Kitty, are counting on twenty volts of electricity to jolt their brains back into equilibrium. Muscle relaxant ensures that the only signal of their seizure will be a twitch of the toe; anesthesia guarantees that they will not remember the paralysis or anything else leading to the convulsion. Scores more line up for similar sessions at two dozen other hospitals across the state. Even at nearby McLean, one of America's most exalted citadels of psychiatry, fifty patients a week are transfused with enough current to kindle a sixty-watt bulb and, if the procedure is true to its well-established form, vanquish the demons of the moment.

In Massachusetts as in the rest of the nation the evidence is unmistakable: ECT is back.

A procedure pioneered in the 1930s that seemed on the edge of extinction just a generation ago is being performed today at medical centers large and small, on patients staying in the hospital and on a growing number who simply show up an hour before treatment and leave an hour after. More than 100,000 Americans a year get ECT for ailments ranging from mania to catatonia, with ten to twenty times that many worldwide. Electroconvulsive therapy is now as ordinary as a hysterectomy and twice as common as knee replacement surgery. And it all is happening just enough out of sight that it has taken many medical professionals by surprise. Madness no more, electric shock is quietly being resurrected as a restorative wonder that someday could rank right up there with penicillin and Prozac.

How one of the most reviled psychiatric procedures is fast becoming one of its mainstays is an astounding yet untold chapter of American medical history. It is a narrative that begins with an epidemic of mental illness that has stubbornly resisted a cure, and a handful of doctors who have equally stubbornly refused to give up on a remedy that most had banished as barbaric. Researchers still have not filled in the puzzle of how or why ECT provides relief, although the proof is compelling that it does, faster and more surely than drugs or talk therapy. Questions also remain about the price shock patients pay in memories lost, in rare cases permanently, and whether such risks can be minimized or eliminated entirely. The rise, fall, and rise again of ECT thus remains an epic without an ending, as practitioners and potential patients alike wait to see if hopes for success are sustained and it can come back all the way.

Barbara Collins-Layton could not wait. Like millions of Americans, the fifty-six-year-old retired banker suffers serious depression, and has since childhood. It is a family trait, as is the mania that comes after. Her bathroom vanity was beginning to look like a pharmacy, stocked with Risperdal, Zyprexa, Lamictal, and other psychotropic drugs that once worked but did no longer. Her desk was cluttered with crumpled bills from therapists. It had gotten to where she would wake in the morning and make a beeline for the living room and her rocking chair. Forward and back. Lean and tilt. All day long for six long weeks. While she rocked, her three-year-old adopted son whispered: "Did I make Mommy sick?" Collins-Layton finally went to her psychiatrist and pleaded, "I can't do this any longer. I can't live in this state of mind." He suggested ECT.

Looking back six years later, Collins-Layton realizes how radical a treatment ECT is. "Was I afraid to get electricity to my brain?" she asks. "Hell yes!" She remembers what it smelled like—"almost like metal"— her first session. She knows there are questions still unanswered, like whether her lost memories will return. "But it made me function again," Collins-Layton explains from her home in Portage, Indiana. "You don't function sitting in a rocking chair. I didn't shower. I couldn't cook. I couldn't take care of my family. It takes awhile with ECT. I had like six treatments. But when I came home from the hospital I was functioning again. ECT gave me my life back."

∽✑

One thing ECT is not is photogenic.

The typical patient looks as grisly as she feels. She has had nothing to drink in two hours, nothing to eat in eight. No hairpins allowed, or jewelry. No hair spray, mousse, eyeglasses, contact lenses, hearing aids, dentures, or anything else that could short-circuit the electrodes or burn the patient. Chewing gum is verboten. So is nail polish, at least on the fingers or toes where doctors will watch for signs of a seizure. There is little sense of self-command as she is rolled in in a wheelchair and lies in wait on a stretcher. Chances are she has come from a locked ward where she has had too much time to ruminate on the impending procedure or, worse still, been briefed by the frazzled soul in the next room.

"I'm sitting in the waiting area and other people there for treatment are watching TV," remembers Barbara, a sixty-six-year-old nun who had a dozen sessions of ECT several years ago at a suburban hospital. She had neither read about the treatment nor seen it in the movies. No one in her closed world of the convent had had it. Nothing had prepared her for the despair. "The nurse comes down and calls the names of five people. Then she calls my name. I nearly died," says Sister Barbara. "People I was going up in the elevator with looked so sick. So sick. I said to myself, 'I'm depressed, but not that sick.' There's a look, there is a way their body operates—someone who walks relatively stiffly, their arms down by their side. They know where they are—on the elevator—but beyond that they don't really know."

ECT's setting does not help. Ordinarily, the procedure is done in the postanesthesia care unit, or PACU, just as the hospital is waking up. Those choices are logical: The PACU has the required curtained cubicle dividers, movable stretchers, highly trained nurses, and medical monitors, and since regular surgeries have barely begun—it's 7:00 a.m.—the recovery unit will be empty for the next hour or two. But the where and when of ECT can also be stigmatizing. Most ECT units are in a secluded section of the hospital, sometimes in the basement. Stainless steel is everywhere. Fluorescent lights. The feel and smell of antiseptics. No soothing paintings here, no racks of magazines or wall-mounted television set, no comfortable chairs standard in obstetrics, gynecology, and other departments where today's spin-savvy hospitals market and define themselves. The remote location does shield patients from running into anyone they know; even better, it makes it unlikely that other patients, staff, or the public will find out that ECT is being done there. Those odds of anonymity are enhanced by scheduling the procedure at a time when most patients and physicians are still eating breakfast.

The treatment cubicle itself is occupied by a medley of wires and electrodes, along with a medical team that vaults into action the instant a patient arrives, a reminder of how many more are waiting and how soon the room will revert to its intended use for surgical recoveries. A nurse takes vital signs. The ECT doc fastens sensors to the stomach, head, limbs, and finger, up to eleven in all. Green, brown, black, red, and white hues tell him which wires go to the machine monitoring heart rate and rhythm, which connect to devices checking brain waves and oxygen levels in the blood. The anesthesiologist inserts a needle in the vein and attaches an intravenous line, standard practice for any procedure requiring anesthesia.

What happens next is aimed at shielding the body from the shock delivered to the brain. A short-acting sleeping medication is injected, and thirty seconds later the patient is out cold. A muscle relaxant is added, producing near-complete paralysis and guarding against the writhing and flailing of the treatment's bad old days. The anesthetic drugs leave the patient unable to breathe on her own, so she is hooked to a supply of pure oxygen that breathes for her and protects her brain. The anesthesiologist inserts a plastic bite-block or cotton cushion in the patient's mouth to keep her from biting her tongue or cracking a tooth, a safeguard that works even better when a doctor or nurse grasps her chin just before the pulse is delivered. Final preparations: parting the hair, cleaning the scalp with rubbing alcohol where two half-dollar-size metal electrodes will go, then applying a conductive gel that makes it easier for the current to make contact with the cranium.

Electricity comes from a wall plug, activates with the push of a button, and is the centerpiece of everything that makes ECT spellbinding as well as odious. A device that looks like a stereo receiver transforms the current into a waveform intended to be safe and therapeutic. A wire and a pair of six-inch electrodes the shape of thread spools connect the ECT machine to the patient's head. The right dose is critical, and most doctors still use a formula based on a patient's age (older means more), sex (men need more), other medications (some impede a convulsion), and how oily the skin and thick the skull are (thicker and oilier call for a higher dose). The energy actually delivered to the brain is less than one amp, or a third of what comes from a cardiac defibrillator and a fraction of the seven amps needed to power a vacuum cleaner.

The aim of that jolt—the holy grail of ECT—is to stimulate a seizure powerful enough to fire off the cells of the brain in rhythmic synchrony. Think of all the lightbulbs in Manhattan flicking on and off, at the same time, several times a second. Or imagine what happens with epilepsy, only there the convulsion is violent, while with electroshock, anesthesia and muscle relaxants ensure the patient is almost motionless. The ECT device shoots its current for at most eight seconds, and often just half a second—so quick it is impossible to track on a watch and so quiet an untrained observer would not know anything was happening if not for three beeps from the machine beforehand. The seizure itself is over in as few as fifteen seconds, and seldom lasts longer than sixty. The patient's jaw may tighten and her face flush slightly when the stimulus is applied, and during the seizure there is a twitch of the toes or fingers. Corroboration of a grand mal seizure comes from three sources: an electrocardiogram that shows a spike in heart rate, an electroencephalogram that reveals changes in the brain's electrical activity, and a blood pressure cuff that reflects an increase in pressure.

The whole routine, from the time a patient counts herself to sleep to when she is moved to the recovery bay, normally takes less than fifteen minutes and is often over in five. That is a good thing, since the process is likely to be repeated six to twelve times in the next two to three weeks—and if that series works, even more shock may be given to prevent symptoms from coming back or battle them when they do.

For Rhoda Falk, the ECT treatments she had in the 1940s and again in the 1960s were painless and successful but invasive enough that she would never do it again. "A procedure like that is like having a cataract operation. When you're older, anything drastic like that you shy away from," says Falk, who is eighty-one and lives in Prescott, Arizona. But fifty-eight-year-old Laurel Zangerl, who had her first ECT ten years ago, says that "with muscle relaxants and anesthesia, you might have a headache after or feel a little groggy, but you don't feel horrible or shocked or anything like that. It's not a wonderfully pleasant experience, but I would rather have ECT than have a tooth pulled by a dentist or a crown replaced. And it definitely is better than root canal."

❧

Researchers have assembled a clear profile of today's ECT patient, and she looks a lot like Geraldine Knaack.

She is the first defining characteristic. More than two out of three ECT patients are women, a trend that holds whether the treatment is being given in Finland or England, New Zealand or, in Knaack's case, Neenah, Wisconsin. The gender difference is not surprising, since nearly twice as many women as men are diagnosed with depression, and depression is the most common condition for which ECT is prescribed. But research also suggests that, for reasons no one has pinned down, doctors may be quicker to prescribe ECT to female patients, who in turn may be quicker to agree.

Knaack's age, sixty-eight, is another giveaway. One national survey showed that more than a third of hospitalized ECT patients are over sixty-five—quadruple their share of the population of psychiatric patients. A poll of New York hospitals found that more than half of ECT recipients were older than sixty. Why the yawning age gap? It is partly that senior citizens suffer more major depression than other age groups, especially if they live in a nursing home, and suicide is much more common among older Americans. Potential interactions with drugs they are taking for medical maladies put the elderly at risk with antidepressants, making them more likely to turn quickly to an alternative like ECT. And an aging population means more Americans meeting those criteria. Insurance plays a role, too, with Medicare helping the elderly afford electroconvulsive treatment, a single session of which adds about $3,000 to a hospital stay and costs up to $2,000 as an outpatient procedure. (A full series, involving six to twelve treatments, costs between $12,000 and $36,000.) ECT critics say seniors are easily coerced into having the treatment, but more convincing is evidence that it works even better for older patients. The National Institutes of Health has concluded that, even with their high use relative to other age groups, for the elderly, ECT "is generally underused or unavailable."

The typical ECT patient also is white, rich, and a Yankee. Few African Americans and Hispanics get it, although no one is sure whether that is because of income, race, or something else. Money is easier to explain: It buys the insurance that pays for ECT, or lets a patient pay out of pocket, and it increases the odds that she will seek treatment for her mental illness. She is more likely to seek that treatment at a private hospital than a government-supported one, to live in an area with lots of psychiatrists and not many legal restrictions on ECT, and to be from the Northeast or Midwest. All of which describes Knaack but belies the public perception of ECT left over from the 1950s and 1960s, when the treatment was rightfully criticized as being used disproportionately on poor wards of state mental asylums.

Today, there is an opposite, equally troubling concern: that the poor are denied ECT. People without private insurance used to be able to get ECT at state hospitals. But since being branded "shock factories" in the 1960s and 1970s, few public facilities are willing to bear the stigma or cost of the treatment. Eighty percent of state hospitals across the South failed to administer a single ECT in 1986—and it was not even an option at the nineteen state hospitals built since 1970, according to a survey published in 1989. The situation probably has worsened since then, with the ranks of the uninsured swelling and public hospitals across the country still wary about electroshock. In Manhattan, for instance, ECT is available at New York University Medical School's upscale Tisch Hospital but not at the NYU-affiliated Bellevue Hospital, which is city-owned and caters to a poorer population. "The reason," says Dr. Jonathan Brodie, interim chairman of psychiatry at NYU, "is grounded only in ignorance and history. Policies at public hospitals are decided by lay boards of directors, who chased ECT out of the public domain. They decided this was a barbaric treatment and now public institutions no longer do it. It means that poor people are denied wonderful care. ECT is a wonderful treatment when it is used appropriately."

What unites ECT patients more than anything is an unrelenting, unbearable sickness.

"It gets to the point where you just do not recognize yourself," Marc Pierre, a physical therapist in Los Angeles, says of the depression he has experienced. "You look in the mirror and just have no connection to what you are seeing. The fire raging inside your skull is so intense and requires so much energy it is difficult to interject any sense of beauty, of appreciation, of love . . . I was heading into the well with no stairway." That is how Pierre felt five years ago, before eight months of ECT. Shock treatment was his safety net. "It pulled me from an abyss of psychological despair," he explains, "towards an actual capability to experience life as a positive force."

Geraldine Knaack's long-suffered depression bottomed out with a "complete nervous breakdown" in 1990. She spent thirty days in the hospital, where "my only recall is walking in the door with my husband. I also remember an incident in lockup where I was screaming, crying, and clawing at my arms until it drew blood. I remember a male nurse telling me to stop or they'd put me in the county home." Drawing blood became a pattern, generally by cutting herself with glass. It was always on the top of her left hand, which is now laced with scars, and she always stopped just short of killing herself. Drinking was another way of crying for help and taming the ogres within. "I had never been much of a drinker," she recalls, "but one night I made myself a rum and Coke. The next night I drank two, the night after that I drank three." The alcohol did not mix well with the twenty-five antidepressants and other pills she took every day, but that did not slow her down. "The next day I drank three again," she says. "I wasn't an alcoholic. I was trying basically to kill myself. I kept making the drinks stronger and stronger." In retrospect, Knaack knows she was nearing the limit, the point where her brain and other organs could no longer absorb the abuse. "If I'd kept on going I probably would have been dead. I *would* have been dead."

Whenever things have gotten really bad, from 1990 until now, Knaack has had a series of ECT treatments. The first set brought her back from her breakdown. Another restored her after nearly a year of mourning for Judy, her identical twin, who died the day Geraldine went into the hospital for open heart surgery in 1996. The illness remains, but electric shock has proven it can banish into remission the crippling symptoms in a way no other therapy can. "The ECTs have literally saved my life, many times. I used to be afraid of them, but not anymore," she says. "Even my husband has come around. He didn't like me having them, but even he has admitted they helped."

Severe depression like Pierre's and Knaack's is the most widespread form of mental illness in America, afflicting some 10 million people a year.* It also is the most common reason people are referred for ECT, accounting for more than 80 percent of use. People with schizophrenia make up fewer than one in ten ECT patients, a dramatic drop-off from the 1930s, when they were its first and most frequent users. That is because society is better at distinguishing real schizophrenia from conditions with equivalent symptoms, and because antipsychotic drugs now are the frontline treatment. The situation is similar with the frenetic talking, thinking, and doing we associate with mania, as well as with alternating highs and lows lumped under the rubric of bipolar disorder. ECT clearly can help, but with the availability of alternatives like lithium, people with mania or bipolar disorder constitute just 3 percent of ECT users. Depressed or otherwise impaired pregnant women use it because they fear that psychotropic drugs might injure their fetuses. And while it has been used effectively and safely by adolescents and children, it seldom is.

Catherine Steinhoff knows that her daughter Katie was not the classic ECT user when she got her first treatment in early 2005. Katie had mania, not depression. She was seventeen, young enough to face legal hurdles to getting ECT in some states and practical ones just about

---

*Adding in less severe depression and bipolar disorder, the number rises to 19 million a year, according to the National Institute of Mental Health. Another NIMH-sponsored survey found that 62 million Americans will suffer some form of depression during their lives.

everywhere. But Catherine also knew that Katie had barely functioned for the previous two years when, without warning, her illness surfaced. "Katie had lost her life in all respects. I think I would have tried voodoo dolls," her mother recalls. "And she ended up getting better immediately after that first treatment. She had nine in all. It's not like it is all gone and she'll never be sick again. Whether it will hold for her we don't know, it's pretty early to be calling this a success. But now something has worked for Katie when nothing had worked for Katie for two years."

Katie admits she was "freaked out" when she was first told about getting ECT. "I just didn't want to do it. It was like, electric shock!" But medicines made her "different" and were not working, so she agreed to try ECT. "Now I'm not manic anymore. I would think people were talking about me, filming me. I had this paranoia. That's gone, or at least I have it only every once in a while now. I feel like it's fixed."

Feeling better has come at a price for Katie, the way it does for most ECT patients. "I don't remember things very easily," she says. "Yesterday I was going to the Taste Buds restaurant. I have been there a million times and I didn't know what it was. When they said, 'We're going to Taste Buds,' I didn't know what they were talking about." With prompting by her mother and others those memories are coming back, and she says that if her condition gets bad again, "I would be totally fine with having ECT again."

❦

Twenty-five years ago ECT seemed on its way to the same dustbin of discredited remedies as mustard plaster, bloodletting, and lobotomies. Screenwriters were taking flights of fantasy to cuckoo's nests, snake pits, and shock corridors. ECT critics—from former patients who felt betrayed and even ruined, to counterculturalists who saw psychiatry and especially electroconvulsive therapy as embodying all they detested in the military-industrial complex—sought to ban or at least discredit it.

Most psychiatrists were willing to give up without a fight, dropping the "dirty drug" of ECT in favor of shelves full of psychopotions and renewed faith in Father Freud. The public, as early as the 1970s, was losing whatever faith it had in such a jolting cure.

Dr. Robert L. Palmer, a prominent British psychiatrist, sounded ECT's death knell in his 1981 book on the treatment: "It is my personal prediction that the widespread practice of ECT will not last for another forty years, nor indeed to the end of the century. Perhaps even by the end of this decade, electroconvulsive therapy for severe depressive states will probably have been replaced by more effective and selective drugs. ECT will pass into history and will be judged in that perspective." A pair of researchers at the National Institute of Mental Health backed up Palmer's intuition with numbers. In just the five years from 1975 to 1980, ECT usage nationwide had tumbled a dramatic 46 percent. At state and county mental hospitals, once the epicenter of electroconvulsion, the decline was a whopping 74 percent and the number of patients treated in 1980 a trifling 1,221.

What Palmer and other prophets of doom could not foresee was that older wonder drugs like Tofranil and newer ones like Prozac would prove a flop, immediately or over time, for about one in five people taking them. Others experienced disquieting side effects: losing their sex drive or prowess, gaining fifty or more pounds, having trouble keeping their heads up during the day or staying asleep at night, or suffering the double whammy of aching stomach and throbbing head. Psychotropics were a boon for millions, and their promise of relief brought millions more under the care of mental health professionals, but drugs were not enough. Patients recognized that, and demanded more. So, eventually, did doctors and the psychiatric establishment. High-powered studies in the late 1970s and 1980s from Britain's Royal College of Psychiatrists and America's National Institutes of Health rallied around electroconvulsive therapy and answered its critics. Most convincing of all, while the limits of other treatments were becoming ever clearer, new and more rigorous research reinforced just how quickly and effectively ECT worked for those patients who were the sickest and most in need of immediate help. The corpse was not quite ready for burial.

One of the two NIMH-supported researchers who had documented ECT's fall from the precipice in 1980 went back to the data and found that, between then and 1986, the slide had leveled off and usage might have risen slightly. Other reports suggested a robust recovery. Doctors also were giving ECT a second look, judging from the near doubling of scientific articles published in the mid-1980s compared to a decade earlier. A survey of Medicare recipients, meanwhile, found that the number getting ECT shot up 30 percent from 1987 to 1992.

Julaine Siegel was one of the faces behind those figures. She had her first ECT in the early 1980s, her second ten years later. "I was not responding to medications. In fact, I was dying," says the fifty-one-year-old therapist. "I would pace the floor nonstop twenty-four hours a day. I tried various medications but they were not helping. The ECT relieved a lot of anxiety and depression within about two weeks. I was not totally well, but I could function. I was eating a little. I stopped pacing. I would not be alive today if I didn't have ECT, plain and simple. It bridged the gap and gave me time to breathe until I could find a medication that worked."

Desperation like that is common enough to continue ECT's rebound into the new millennium, even in the epicenter of anti-ECT America. Consider the evidence from California, which requires every hospital to report every procedure performed and was one of the first states to clamp down on the use of electric shock. It is prescribed only a third as often there as in the rest of the country, studies suggest, but that has been true for more than thirty years. More surprising is the trend within the state: From 1977, the first year reporting was required, through 1994, the numbers of ECT patients went up and down with no pattern. Since then, there has been a clear if not entirely consistent increase, with the 3,498 patients treated in 2003 reflecting a 38 percent jump from 1994 and 44 percent since 1977.

The pattern in Texas, where restrictive regulations took effect twenty years after California's, is similar. The number of ECT patients initially plummeted, hitting a low of 1,454 in 2001. But two years later they were back up by 14 percent, to 1,656. In Vermont, one of a handful of other states with rigorous reporting requirements, there has been a steady rise since state officials began tracking cases during the summer of 2000.

Buried in raw data like that are two striking shifts in the way ECT is used. The first has to do with *when* the treatment is called upon. In its halcyon days from the 1940s through the 1960s, it was a frontline, first-resort therapy. Today, it generally is a last resort, used only after drugs, psychotherapy, and other alternatives have failed. That is logical, given the availability of new antidepressants and other psychotropic medicines and the fact that ECT is an intrusive procedure. It is also a carryover of fears and prejudices and has many practitioners weighing whether it ought to be used earlier for certain groups of patients.

The second change is a matter of *where*. ECT is done on an outpatient basis much more often than it was forty years ago, or even twenty. That growth has been fueled in part by managed-care companies' obsession with keeping down costs, in this case by eliminating hospital charges. Most patients understandably prefer not to stay in the hospital, especially if that means being in a locked psychiatric ward. Doctors generally are willing for patients to head home after treatment provided they are not suicidal, do not have major medical complications, and have someone to drive them home and care for them there. The result is that, like Kitty Dukakis, a third of ECT patients today are in and out of the hospital in under two hours. With that greater ease comes greater use.

So how many Americans are getting ECT today? The studies are better at picking up trends than pinning down numbers. Some review psychiatric hospital records. Others poll psychiatrists. All extrapolate from small samples and are subject to doctors' and patients' understandable reluctance to share information about such a controversial procedure. Even with those caveats, certain trends are clear: ECT use was highest in the 1950s and 1960s, with as many as 300,000 patients a year getting the procedure. The practice plummeted from the mid-1970s to the mid-1980s, then began a slow climb back.

Today, the number of Americans getting ECT each year is about 100,000 and growing.

ECT's fate worldwide mirrors that in the United States. A handful of countries have been even more hell-bent against ECT than states like Texas and California. Slovenia outlawed it in 1994. Italy, which gave birth to the procedure in 1938, sixty years later set limits so strict they amounted to a ban. It has been eradicated from certain cantons in Switzerland and is difficult to get in the European capital of Brussels as well as in Germany and Holland. The antipathy sometimes grew out of politics, the way it did in Italy, where ECT was the symbol of psychiatric authority back in 1978 when the country was swept up in a demedicalized, community-based mental health movement. In Germany the driving force was history, and a recollection that shock was part of the medical experiments the Nazis ran on unwitting, unwilling victims.

In England, which traditionally was second only to the United States in its enthusiasm for ECT, use plummeted the same way it had in America, although the drop came a decade later. The number of treatments given across England in 1999 was fewer than half those administered in 1985. In Scandinavia, by contrast, ECT remains widely available and popular, especially in Sweden, Denmark, and Norway, where it holds an equal footing with psychotherapy and psychopharmacology. "Very hostile anti-ECT sentiments have not been able to gain access to the public mind here," explains Dr. Tom G. Bolwig, professor of psychiatry at the University of Copenhagen and Denmark's leading ECT researcher. "That's partly because in Scandinavia people are a little bit skeptical. If critics are too dramatic, people say, 'Come on.' People seem to have trust in the psychiatric system. And I can definitely say that if I get psychotic depression, I hope someone would be merciful enough to give me ECT."

The largest number of ECT patients is in the Third World. The allure there is its low cost and high success rate, but there is nothing alluring about the way it is administered. In Nigeria, for example, ECT is widely used, for schizophrenia as well as depression, and it is almost always given without anesthesia or muscle relaxants, the way it was in the earliest days in Rome and New York. Cost is the key. The poor African nation cannot afford the psychiatrists or anesthesiologists who administer ECT in the West, or the medicines they use, so it relies on psychiatric nurses and patients' tolerance for pain. Researchers say they have found no evidence of physical damage to people who get Nigerian-style ECT; they say nothing about emotional effects.

Nigeria is not alone. Reports of ECT without anesthesia and muscle relaxants still pour in from Russia, Thailand, Japan, and other countries. In India, a 2002 survey found that even in teaching hospitals, more than half the patients get ECT without benefit of anesthesia, and a full third are being treated for schizophrenia, a condition where its use as a frontline treatment is questionable.* In Thailand, 94 percent get ECT without anesthesia, and 74 percent get it to relieve schizophrenia. The situation is similar in China, where some doctors blend Eastern medicine with Western by applying the electrodes to the same spots on the head where they would put acupuncture needles. In Turkey, ECT is used in its raw form on psychiatric patients as young as nine, with nothing to dull the pain, a human rights group reports. It also allegedly is employed as punishment, with patients dragged to treatment in straitjackets. The highest rate of usage in the world may be in Nepal, where ECT is

---

*India has only 4,000 psychiatrists for its population of 1 billion, compared with 40,000 for 300 million Americans, and it spends a fraction of the money on mental health. Ironically, as India moves to beef up its psychiatric services, some psychiatrists there question whether ECT still has a role. In the United States and other countries that India is trying to emulate, much of the public sees ECT as backward if not barbaric, these Indian psychiatrists argue, so India should give up the therapy if it wants to polish its image.

given to one in four psychiatric hospital patients, six times the rate in the United States.

Adding up the numbers of patients treated and procedures performed is even more difficult internationally than for America, because there are few studies being conducted outside Europe, and reports from China, India, and Africa are sketchy. One U.S. expert, recently back from training his counterparts in China, says that more than 1 million Chinese get ECT annually, with at least that many in India. Others say it is far fewer, although growing fast. The best estimate worldwide is that 2 million people are treated every year, receiving more than 15 million sessions of shock therapy.

ECT's rebound is radical, although not without precedent. The first human heart transplant was performed with enormous fanfare in 1967 by South Africa's Dr. Christiaan Barnard, but by 1971 the surgery seemed cursed, with nearly every recipient having died. Thanks to the persistence of surgeons who believed in it, and the discovery of a drug that suppresses organ rejection without knocking out the body's natural defenses, the operation rebounded to the point where today more than two thousand Americans a year are kept alive with transplanted hearts. Smallpox vaccinations are another case where a treatment was delayed if not doomed, in this case by opposition to compulsory immunization in the 1890s that boiled over into riots from Montreal to Milwaukee. Then there are folk remedies like leeches, which were used for twenty-five hundred years to treat everything from headaches to stomachaches, then discarded as primitive if not putrefying. Today the bloodsucking crawlers are back in operating rooms, battling clots and removing congested corpuscles from wounds.

But with transplants, leeches, and most other therapies that have bounced back, the recovery was impossible to miss for anyone paying attention, and certainly for the medical community and media. ECT is different. Its turnaround has happened sub rosa, with no acknowledgment from the public and little from the press. A 1990 *San Francisco Bay Guardian* headline announced "Electroshock's Quiet Comeback," noting that ECT's return to local hospitals was "shrouded in secrecy." The announcement itself was secreted back on page seventeen. Four months later, headline writers at the *New York Times* chose nearly identical words—and a similarly remote location, page seven of the science section—to discuss the "Quiet Comeback of Electroshock Therapy." Which is just the low profile most patients and doctors wanted, at least until recently.

Silence is an old story for the mentally ill. Most would not hesitate to tell family, friends, and even bosses, if they had cancer or diabetes. Yet they rightfully worry about being branded defective if they admit being mired in depression, on a manic high, or, worse still, listening to voices that only a schizophrenic can hear. While understanding about mental illness is on the rise, the shame remains when the preferred treatment is ECT.

ECT patients have put a name to their quandary: double stigma. "I feel doubly stigmatized by having been mentally ill and by having had ECT," explains Joyce Jackson, a nurse who had the treatment twice, in 1982 and 1986. "So, except for two trusted friends, I have kept my ECT history a secret." Marie DeRose, also a nurse, chose not to keep secret the ECT she got in 1967, and it "cost me a job" at the adolescent unit of a Boston hospital. Eighteen years later, working in the adult psychiatric unit at the same hospital, DeRose ended up talking to one of the people who had refused to hire her. "She said, 'Well, we were afraid you were too open about your ECT and you might not work well on our team,'" DeRose recalls. "That was ridiculous. If anything, my experience would have been a way to help me understand those patients." Rosemary Goodwin, who is fifty-two and lives in Tewksbury, Massachusetts, says she never broadcast that she had ECT. She did not tell friends, relatives, neighbors, or anyone else. "I didn't want anyone knowing I was a crazy lady," Goodwin says. "When they hear you had shock treatment they think you're way off."

But ECT patients like Goodwin are starting to stand up and talk back. They are tired of only the critics giving voice to what ECT is like, and call themselves the silent majority. The image they identify with is not the crazy aunt in the attic but with blacks who balked at giving up their bus seats to whites, gays suffocating in the closet, and the mentally ill who insist their illness is as real and disabling as any physical one. For Jackson, that meant writing an article, entitled "Electroconvulsive Therapy: Problems and Prejudices." For Goodwin and DeRose, it meant agreeing to be named in this book, although in DeRose's case she asked that it be her maiden name.

Psychologist Martha Manning vents her frustration with ECT's stigma in *Undercurrents,* her critically acclaimed book published in 1994. "For months, in my conversations with most people, I have glossed over ECT's contribution to the end of my depression. But lately I've been thinking, 'Damn it. I didn't rob a bank. I didn't kill anybody. I have nothing to be ashamed of.' I've started telling people about the ECT," she writes. "My admission is typically met with uncomfortable silences and abrupt shifts in topic. An acquaintance at a party is outraged. 'How could you let them do that to you?' I bristle and answer, 'I didn't let them do it to me. I asked them to do it.'" Her first talk after the book came out was at Smith College, she recalls, and "as my escort was bringing me closer, I saw that people were there already. The escort said, 'People are protesting, there must be two speeches there.' But I could see the protest was against me." Manning was experiencing the same thing others have, before and since, who stood up in favor of ECT: a thundering backlash from anti-ECT activists. "It was just the strangest experience. I got in there and this woman gives me a [verbal] punch-out like you wouldn't believe. Then through the tour they added a little security for me."

Voices like Manning's and Jackson's are amplified by celebrities who have gone public with their ECT experiences, a trend that has helped demystify the treatment and stoke its rebound. TV talk-show host Dick Cavett told *People* magazine that for him, ECT was "like a magic wand." Patty Duke, star of Broadway, television, and film, wrote in her memoir on bipolar disorder that "not only does ECT reverse serious depression quickly, it may work for out-of-control mania." Pianist Vladimir Horowitz has made known his positive experience with shock treatment, while Roland Kohloff, principal timpanist for the New York Philharmonic, told the *New York Times* that "what I think it did was to act like a Roto-Rooter on the depression." Dr. Leon Rosenberg, former dean of the Yale Medical School and former ECT patient, has written a magazine article about his "life-saving" experience and given talks on it to medical students and doctors. His message is simple: "It ought not to be a whispered approach to a dread disease."

∽∾

ECT's comeback is not complete. There are still too many impassioned critics who make too many legitimate points. Their main objection is that ECT causes memory loss, which it can, although there is fiery debate over how often, how much, and for how long. Memory problems are worse than most ECT doctors acknowledge but not as bad as many critics charge. More can and is being done to limit the loss. Opponents also insist that ECT causes brain damage. There *is* compelling evidence that ECT changes brain chemistry but little proof that that amounts to damage. The changes may actually be beneficial, at least in the short run.

Outside critics are not the only ones laying siege to ECT: The treatment remains a stepchild within the psychiatric profession. You can measure that second-class status in the scarcity of research funds, from government or industry, devoted to answering nagging questions about the right spot on the scalp to apply electrodes or the best way to safeguard a patient's memory. You can hear it in the reluctance of psychopharmacologists and psychoanalysts to recommend ECT to patients who are not getting better with drugs or talk therapy. You can sense it in the way psychiatric departments bury their ECT clinics in out-of-the-way areas of the hospital, entrust them to junior staff, and wheel them out only at the eleventh hour.

"The attitude toward ECT displayed by many teaching psychiatrists and psychoanalysts varied from overt antagonism to smug condescension," Dr. Zigmond M. Lebensohn, an ECT pioneer and former chief of psychiatry at Sibley Memorial Hospital in Washington, D.C., wrote several years ago in a psychiatric journal. "The psychiatrist who still administered ECT was often viewed with the same gaze that gynecologists used to reserve for their colleagues who performed abortions in the days before legalization. In some centers, a double standard seemed to exist. I have known analysts who condemn ECT in public but who have privately recommended it for individual patients and even for members of their own family."

Dr. Elizabeth Childs, who ran the ECT program at Boston's Carney Hospital before taking over in 2003 as commissioner of mental health for Massachusetts, says that whenever she raises the ECT option with fellow psychiatrists, "they say, 'There you go again.' They think of me as a cowboy because I talk about ECT." Childs thinks psychiatrists' reluctance to consider ECT stems from more than prejudice or fear. "It's a very deep cultural thing in our profession that we still doubt the true pain of mental illness, and we as physicians give up. We don't believe in the resiliency of human beings to get better. We've got to say, 'I'm willing to bring to bear everything in my armamentarium to get them better.' If you don't believe someone really is ill, you aren't going to take a chance with a procedure like ECT. If you don't believe they are going to get better then you won't be willing to expose a patient to ECT's side effects, and it does have significant side effects."

Whatever the reason, the result of psychiatry's qualms about ECT is that too few young psychiatrists are being trained to perform the complicated procedure—fewer still to believe in it. In a 1987 survey, chiefs of psychiatric training programs ranked ECT forty-second among forty-eight skills critical for psychiatrists, putting it barely ahead of play therapy and well behind prescribing drugs and getting along with nurses and social workers. Another survey, published in 1998 by researchers at Harvard, found that fewer than 8 percent of U.S. psychiatrists provide ECT. Who are those rare few? They are more likely to have been trained in a medical school outside the United States, and to have gotten that training in the 1960s or 1980s rather than the anti-ECT era of the 1970s. They also focus their practice on drugs more than therapy, practice at private rather than county or state hospitals, and for the most part are male.

"Most residents get some exposure to ECT, but in most cases the exposure is very, very limited," says Dr. Richard Weiner of Duke University, who runs what may be the world's most esteemed ECT training program. "Residency review committees say that residents have to have an understanding of ECT—its indications, benefits, and risks. But the committees don't say that residents have to be competent to administer ECT."

Medical students are even less likely to know anything about ECT, and their conceptions are often even more wild-eyed and wrong-headed than the public's. A recent survey of students at the University of Arkansas for Medical Sciences found that few knew any technical details of the treatment, including that it was done under general anesthesia. Thirty-one percent thought it was used to punish violent or uncooperative patients, 30 percent believed it was used more often on the poor and minorities, and 24 percent said it causes brain damage. None of which is surprising, since these young people's primary source of information was the movies.

It is not just the young who are at a loss. There is no national requirement that older psychiatrists be recertified in the latest techniques, which is especially important in a field like ECT, where the state of the art is perpetually shifting. Even back when they began practice, no proof was required that they knew the ins and outs of the technology. Many ECT doctors do sign up for retraining, at Weiner's program at Duke or the annual one-day session run by the Association of Convulsive Therapy, but they do so at their own initiative or at the insistence of their hospital. This failure to keep up, the Harvard researchers found, was a key reason why psychiatrists who graduated from medical school between 1940 and 1960

were eight times more likely than newly trained psychiatrists to use ECT
for inappropriate diagnoses, while those graduating from 1961 to 1980
were five times more likely.

Concerns like those led Childs to shut down the ECT program at
Carney Hospital in Boston just three months after she took it over in
1996. "We had to retrain and retool the staff so they were more updated
in their approach. The consent process needed to be clearer and better,
really making sure that patients were competent to consent to the treatment," she recalls. Carney contracted with Beth Israel Deaconess Medical Center, a nearby Harvard teaching hospital, to retrain its ECT staff.
It replaced its ECT machine with a more up-to-date model. And it set
tight criteria limiting when ECT could be used and requiring a second
medical opinion for patients who did not meet those guidelines.

"If Carney needed to retool, that has to be the case at other institutions," adds Childs who, in her current job as mental health commissioner, oversees all thirty Massachusetts hospitals licensed to administer
ECT. "It's not that we at Carney were unique."

Such training gaps help explain why high-quality ECT is out of reach
to so many patients in so much of America. If you happen to live near
the Mayo Clinic in Minnesota, University of Michigan in Ann Arbor, or
University of Virginia in Charlottesville, you have easy access to first-rate
ECT. But live in parts of California or the backwaters of Louisiana, and
just finding a doctor who performs it is nigh impossible. No ECT is
done in a third of American cities; in the rest, usage rates vary dramatically, with hospitals in some communities administering it five times as
often as in others. Grandparents are nearly seven times more likely to get
it than their children, and their grandchildren are almost sure not to even
have heard about it, though it could help them just as much. If today's
typical ECT recipient is rich, white, and old, the patient most likely to
be denied treatment in America is poor, black, and under eighteen.

Limits like those are one of many signs that even with its rising use,

ECT is not nearly as widespread as it could and some say should be. Consider that 20 percent of Americans who suffer serious depression—some 4 million people—do not respond to antidepressant medications or cannot tolerate the side effects. Rather than asking why as many as 100,000 patients get ECT each year in the United States, the question may be why more of those 4 million who are desperate for a remedy are not trying electric shock.

As unsettling as the gaps in access are, even worse is that when it is tapped, ECT too often is used clumsily. A review of New York area hospitals by researchers at Columbia University found that some facilities take steps to limit and measure memory loss, but others do not. Most use EEGs and other high-tech equipment to monitor seizures, but some do not. Those and other deviations from recommended practices "raise public health concerns," the authors said, enough so that they went back for a deeper look. The results, again, were disturbing: ECT worked only half as well in the community hospitals where most patients are treated, compared to academic medical centers where most studies on its effectiveness are run. Sometimes that was because doctors stopped treatment too early. Often they did not ensure enough follow-up therapy. The problem, the authors concluded, was not the ECT itself, but the way it was being administered.

Variation is common in the medical world, where university researchers often have an edge over in-the-trenches physicians on everything from timeliness of training to cutting-edge equipment. But with ECT it is colossally worse, says Dr. Richard Hermann of the Harvard School of Public Health, who has reviewed more ECT usage patterns than any other researcher. "There are things where doctors agree and there is no variation, like hernia repairs," Hermann explains. "There are procedures like appendicitis and tonsillectomy, where there is widespread disagreement. And there is ECT, where frankly there is off-the-charts variation."

The United States is not the only place where ECT is used too little and too unevenly. In Ireland, some hospitals administer ECT twenty-two times more often than others, while in Scotland they fluctuate by a factor of eighteen. The Swedes use it at a rate twice that of their Finnish neighbors; Danes do it nearly fifty times more often than Germans. The Third World is even more of a patchwork, with some countries considering it state of the art and others never considering it at all. In England, meanwhile, there are twelvefold differences across health districts, nearly half of hospitals use outdated machines, and far too many ECT doctors are junior trainees who are poorly supervised.

Those findings prompted a stinging editorial in Britain's leading medical journal, *The Lancet.* While it was written a generation ago, three thousand miles from these shores, its message applies equally to today and to the United States, and sets out the challenge facing electroconvulsive therapy as it seeks to complete its turnaround. "If ECT is ever legislated against or falls into disuse," the editorialists warn, "it will not be because it is an ineffective or dangerous treatment; it will be because psychiatrists have failed to supervise and monitor its use adequately. It is not ECT which has brought psychiatry into disrepute. Psychiatry has done just that for ECT."

Three

A DARK PLACE

Diet pills were the first of my addictions and afflictions, and they are the first link in explaining why I am here in the cold, stark recesses of Massachusetts General Hospital, waiting for doctors to infuse my brain with twenty volts of electric current. My fixation with food traces back to 1954 and my senior year at Brookline High, when I started putting on weight and went from a size six to a ten. My mother preached that you can never have too much money or too little body fat. I thought that was shallow but she *was* my mother, and while I resisted the money part I subconsciously accepted her premise that thin is beautiful. Weight resurfaced as an issue my freshman year at Penn State University. I weighed in at 130 pounds, which, at five feet six inches, made me feel like a blob. That old size ten now was trying to squeeze into a twelve, and my mother would welcome me home with, "Kitty, you get fatter and fatter."

I eventually resolved to do what Mother did. I had seen pills in her dressing room and wondered what they were. "Diet pills,

Kitty," she answered. One morning during my junior year in college I searched through her dresser and took a pill, without asking or telling her. It felt good—enough so that I did it again the next morning. Everyone was taking them in the 1950s, even my little sister Jinny. Being thin was everything. We never thought of them by their technical name, amphetamines, or their street names, speed or uppers. Diet pill was a more comforting label, and one that better reflected our naïveté about the danger. In my case, dieting by swallowing a tablet was a way to quickly lose some weight before I got married the first time, to John Chaffetz. I took Mother's pills initially, then when John and I lived on his air force base, military doctors prescribed them. I would take a pill when I woke up, and the feeling of energy lasted the entire day. Mother was concerned, but only about my acting out. "Stop taking them, Kitty," she warned. "You're talking too much." The advice seemed halfhearted if not hypocritical since she was ingesting the same pills. Not only was she hooked on amphetamines, she popped the narcotic painkillers Darvon and Darvocet like they were candy. As for me, I only took one little pill every morning, first Dexedrine, then Syndrox, then others whose names I can't remember but that delivered the same punch. They were all alike to me, and I always stopped with one. And they worked: I weighed 108 pounds when I was married, effortlessly slipping into a size four.

In 1961, John and I divorced, and I headed home from California with our three-year-old son, also named John. I was twenty-four then, and about to start over. I took just one thing back to Boston that I had begun our marriage with four years earlier: my amphetamine habit. The same Boston doctor who had prescribed diet pills to my mother gave them to me. I was taking them when little John and I moved into a bungalow in the Berkshires that first summer after the divorce. I was on them when I met Michael, not long after I got to Boston, and when we got married two years later. I took them before the American Medical Association warned in the late 1960s that ongoing use of diet pills amounted to substance abuse—and afterward. I took them through all three pregnancies with my three kids, and through four miscarriages, which might have been related to the pills. My doctors said not a word. Nada. I think of them as enablers. They had to have suspected the pills were dangerous even before the AMA made it official, and certainly were aware subsequently. I was addicted to amphetamines for a full twenty-six years.

For the first eighteen of those years no one knew. Then in 1974, shortly before his inauguration for the first of three terms as governor, Michael discovered a store of pills in my bureau drawer. I don't know why he was looking—he was no snoop. Part of me wishes he had been, and had uncovered my stash years before. He immediately asked what was going on. Was I all right? I told him the truth: They were to control my weight. I said I'd stop if it would make him feel better. Media pundits would later upbraid him for being so blind for so long. But how could he have known? I was acting the same way I did when we met and married. Yes, I was somewhat erratic and volatile, as always. Why suspect it was drugs that gave me my endless energy? It wasn't as if he hadn't challenged me on my volcanic personality. He would sometimes go for a day or more without speaking to me after I flew off the handle. He can be naïve about emotional issues, and was when he first sensed my drug dependence, but over time he learned, and that first time was not his fault.

Once he knew, Michael insisted I see our family doctor, who got me to lay off the pills. What started me taking them again a few months later? It could have been anything. I was a powder keg ready to explode. I neither asked for nor received help from anyone. I was back on pills and back keeping them secret from my husband. That's the way addicts are. We don't consider it deceit, just getting by. For eight more years I began every day with a synthetic pick-me-up. I don't know what crack cocaine is like, but I had what I suspect were some of the same feelings, feelings of energy that could keep me going for hours and hours. When I erupted, my sister Jinny wrote it off as my being "argumentative." My kids said, "Mommy is in one of her bad moods." Michael called it "Kitty being Kitty." In reality, it was Kitty being a substance abuser.

Like a drug addict, I paid a price for my highs and my cunning. The first time I sneaked a diet pill from Mother's dresser I felt guilty. That feeling persisted each and every day I took another. The drugs cast a shadow over everything. I had gone to college, gotten married, and had a wonderful son. I got divorced, went back to college, earned a bachelor's degree, married again, had two terrific daughters, taught modern dance, and, as the wife of the governor, became involved in all sorts of social programs. I was a founding member of the U.S. Holocaust Memorial Council. I was a founder and president of the Island of Hope program on childhood cancer. I started Massachusetts's Open Space Beautification Program. And you know what? I took no credit for any of that because, deep down, I was sure that everything I had accomplished derived from the pills. No matter how much I did or how many kudos came my way, I had an unshakable sense that I was fooling people.

And I was. I regularly switched pharmacies to fill prescriptions, trying not to tip off anyone about how often I was using. I learned to sniff out physicians and pharmacists who would prescribe without interrogating me. Few really tried. You cannot behave like this without realizing you are being bad. I was living what was in effect a double life—a double lie—conning my husband as well as myself.

It actually was a quadruple lie. I was deceiving Michael and myself not just about my addiction to diet pills but about an equally
disabling one to alcohol. It, too, started half a century ago, during my senior year in high school. I was in charge of Class Day
and had spent the day before getting ready. I was too busy to stop
for lunch. That night friends and I were headed to an event I had
put together called Brookline Night at the Boston Pops. On the
way, we stopped at a party where everyone was drinking punch
laced with alcohol. I had two glasses—a recipe, on my empty
stomach, for retching. Worse than the upset stomach was my embarrassment at having my father, who conducted the Pops and
played first violin for the Boston Symphony, see me in such a
pitiable condition. Strong coffee made me a bit more presentable
as we arrived at our special table at Symphony Hall. For more
than 120 years Boston Symphony musicians have offered up show
tunes, rhapsodies, and other light fare that they call Pops, and one
of the favorite encore numbers when I was in high school was
LeRoy Anderson's "The Waltzing Cat." Large placards introduced the songs. That night the printed announcement for the
Anderson piece got the audience roaring. To honor me, Dad had
changed the title to "The Waltzing Kitty." "The Wobbling Kitty"
would have been more appropriate.

My second drinking episode happened during my sophomore
year at Penn State. I partook of a proud tradition at fraternity parties: having several too many. The result was the same as before:
vomiting. I was mortified enough that I didn't do it again, but not
enough to consider the dangers of drinking or my special vulnerability.

Over my adult years I gradually came to accept that I had a serious problem with drugs. My self-awareness about drinking took longer. I had only been truly drunk three or four times. Hardly the profile of an alcoholic, or so I told myself. Fact was, I drank daily. Every night I had a full shot of vodka. And there were other signs. I was a regular at Boston Pops concerts when my dad was conducting. Seats on the main floor are replaced by tables and chairs when Pops replaces the straiterlaced symphony. Light drinks and snacks are served while the orchestra plays. (The Pops actually got its name from the sound of champagne being uncorked.) I typically hosted two tables and ordered drinks and food. I inevitably finished my sparkling Burgundy before anyone else, then scoped out my guests' glasses. If any wine remained, I secretly fumed. I was ready for more and couldn't understand why they couldn't keep up. Classic alcoholic thinking.

When Michael was reelected as governor in 1982, I was off the diet pills and had stopped drinking. But four months into his second term I was back into the bottle. The drinking I did then was what I termed "under control," which meant not every day and nothing stronger than wine. I know now that alcohol is alcohol is alcohol, whether it is in wine, beer, or spirits. All are equal-opportunity poisons and feed a habit like mine. However much I pretended to be in control, I was not.

Alcohol left me less uplifted than amphetamines, more numb than highly charged. It would be easy to blame the drinking on the stress of being the governor's wife, which was considerable. But I had gotten used to that pressure by the time Michael began serving his third term in 1987. What I was not ready for was the stress that would come a year later with his bid for the White House. Initially, I was buoyed by the excitement. Then, with no warning, I froze. It was just before the New Hampshire primary, and I was petrified at the prospect of his winning the Democratic nomination, not to mention the presidency. I wanted him to win, yet the possibility terrified me. I would be on the road campaigning for a week, then return home to an empty house. With Michael and the children on their own campaign trips, I sat by myself, waiting and worrying. Michael was good enough to be president, but would I be a worthy first lady? Could I withstand the scrutiny of a presidential campaign, which was a hundred times more intense and invasive than stumping for governor? I was one of the first to push him to run. Now I wondered whether I should have. Should I have raised doubts along with hopes? Was I merely an afterthought with my famous husband, same as I had been with my famous father?

I was exhausted from campaigning and certain I was about to embarrass my husband and children. I was lonely and frightened that I couldn't measure up, so I measured out the vodka. Enough, this time, to send me into a stupor. I had commitments, campaign appearances, but they were out of the question in my condition. I canceled two trips before the important Ohio primary and told my staff I had the flu. People were upset at the last-minute no-shows, but they gave me the benefit of their doubts. I didn't give a damn. When Michael came home I was in bed and completely out of it. He was appalled. "Kitty," he asked, "why are you doing this?" I said, "I'll be okay, don't worry." He was too busy with the campaign to see how deep I had fallen. I was too much in denial. I was also a convincing liar.

I bounced back during the fall general election campaign, even as Michael's prospects were faltering. I learned to do my drinking mainly in my head. During the long hours between campaign stops, I would anticipate that sweet cocktail when the day's politicking was done. I pictured it being poured, heard the ice cubes clinking, felt the cool liquid easing down my throat. My staff began to leave a bottle of Stolichnaya in my hotel suite every night.

After everyone was gone, I brought that bottle to bed. I poured myself a shot, draining it a second later, then put the bottle back where they had left it. Anyone paying attention could have seen my trail of three-quarters-full vodka bottles; everyone was too busy to notice. Thank God for my structured days and the campaign's perpetual motion. They were what kept me from turning that single drink into a succession, emptying the bottle rather than leaving it mostly full. Paul Costello, my press secretary then and friend ever since, said it was a shock to find out I had been abusing alcohol, given the late nights and early mornings when I had to be—and was—on my game. He says I was a "functioning alcoholic," which I was. For years I had lived with the guilt of taking diet pills. By the end of the presidential campaign I could hear a similar small voice warning me about my drinking.

The day after the 1988 election, November 9, my staff threw a party for everyone we worked with through the long campaign. The next day I began binge drinking. I made furtive bids to return to work. I went to the State House, where Michael was digging in again, and puttered around aimlessly until I could justify heading home for a drink. Once I was so anxious to get home that I was pulled over for speeding. The officer asked what the hurry was. I could hardly tell him it was my craving for booze. After awhile I stopped showing up at my office. I spent all day at our duplex on Perry Street in Brookline. I got up in the morning, waited for Michael to leave, then canceled all my appointments. I headed straight to the liquor cabinet in the dining room, carried the bottle into the kitchen, poured out three or four ounces of spirits, and gulped it down. Then I grabbed a newspaper or magazine, went upstairs, drew the blinds, unplugged the phone, and read for the ten minutes it took me to pass out. When I got up two hours later, I did it all again. If I had somewhere to go at night, I had my last drink at 2:30 in the afternoon.

At that time in my life a pattern was emerging, one where each episode was a bit worse, a bit more desperate. In December 1988, I invited my neighbors to dinner. Afterward I went into the kitchen to clean up, and proceeded to drink whatever wine was left out of every glass. By the end of that year I no longer stopped drinking in the afternoon, and no longer limited myself to the vodka I preferred. When it ran out, I switched to gin. When the gin was gone, I turned to scotch, then bourbon, and finally brandy. It didn't matter what I was drinking as long as I reached the sought-after status—oblivion. I drank straight, too. No water. No ice. No restraint.

To cover up the stench, I took baths all the time, brushed my teeth a hundred times a day, and ate foods I thought disguised odors. For a while I tried peanut butter, which my sorority sisters at Penn State had used to deceive our housemother, who was president of the local Women's Christian Temperance Union. Altoids and mints worked better. It didn't take long for Michael to catch on. Although he was bombarded by the fragrance of toothpaste and mouthwash, he could sniff through it to detect the scotch and bourbon.

Then came the horrifying incident where my son John found me out cold in my room, lying in a puddle of vomit. Michael rushed home. He washed and cleaned me. Could I humiliate myself any further? I answered my own question in November 1989, the one-year anniversary of Michael's presidential defeat. I was having more than my normal trouble falling asleep. I went into the bathroom and opened the cabinet under the sink. The house had been stripped of dangerous substances, but I spotted a bottle with "alcohol" written near the top. "Rubbing" was right above it, and I saw that, too. I knew rubbing alcohol was different from the drinking kind, but I didn't know how toxic it was. I had no intent to kill myself, I just needed to sleep for a while. I took a small gulp.

I could see myself in the mirror over the sink. It was eerie, like watching myself on television. The alcohol tasted horrible, like fire. I tilted the bottle back and took another swig. Flame on flame. I fumbled my way back to bed. That's all I remember. The obliteration I prized enough to break my sobriety enveloped me. Michael noticed I was breathing funny. He couldn't wake me. He called our family physician, who tried to rouse me, then called for help. Around nine that evening I was taken by ambulance to Brigham and Women's Hospital.

I survived, again, and learned a lesson. Next time I hit bottom I steered clear of rubbing alcohol, opting instead for mouthwash, aftershave, and, of all things, nail polish remover. I didn't take enough of anything for it to show up in my urine test. The time after that I rifled through the house checking every container for alcohol. The vanilla extract had some but not enough. The last thing I swallowed was hair spray. I pulled off the spray nozzle and began gulping. Not knowing what to do this time, Michael summoned my sister and told her to bring a bottle. Anything, even liquor, was safer than hair spray and rubbing alcohol. Jinny was as distraught as Michael. After she left I began to drink. When I awoke the next morning, I started again—drink after drink after drink. This time I did not unplug the phone, and later that day Michael called from the State House. I don't remember the call; it was my first complete blackout. He came home and yet again found me passed out in my own vomit.

As I look back, I see how fortunate I was. I hit bottom relatively quickly. Maybe my addiction to amphetamines had quickened the pace. I have met many recovering alcoholics with painful histories of drinking for twenty-five years or longer. I could not have continued like that for any length of time. My binges were never intended to be suicidal. I just wanted relief. But my behavior was suicidal, it was life-threatening. If I had continued drinking for much longer I would have died.

❧

The alcohol and even the diet pills were symptoms of a deeper-seated affliction: depression.

I suspect the depression was always there, but the amphetamines masked it. How else to interpret the fact that my depression first surfaced in 1982, just after I stopped taking diet pills? Doctors have told me that amphetamines were once used to treat depression, and I may have been treating mine without realizing it. Another possibility is that the pills ignited the depression, the way they do with lots of longtime users of speed who go cold turkey the way I did. In either case the link between getting off drugs and into melancholy makes sense. I am convinced I would have recognized the depression earlier if I hadn't been taking the pills. I certainly had plenty of reason to be depressed earlier in life, whether it was getting divorced or showing up back on my parents' doorstep with my young son. But none of us in those days was terribly sensitive to the whole meaning of depression. And I never felt in despair, or never acknowledged it, until I stopped the amphetamines.

Still more certain is that the depressions I began to experience were related to my drinking. I am not sure which came first, the alcoholism or the depression, but I am sure they are connected. Maureen McGlame, my friend who is a recovery specialist, says I drank as a way of medicating myself and covering up my pain. "You were like a squirrel in a cage," she adds, "going round and round and round." Deprived of that medication, I got out of the cage but fell into despondency. Or maybe the hopelessness was always there, as Maureen says, and the alcohol had numbed it into submission.

Everyone in my family has a different way of detecting when my depression is settling in. To John, it is when I don't want to come to the phone, or stay in bed much of the day. Our daughter Andrea applies the "voice test." I go from sounding animated to sounding emotionally dead, from gushing about everything happening in my world to asking rote questions about hers and not really listening to the answers. Kara, my youngest, remembers coming home from high school and instinctively glancing up at Michael's and my bedroom window before she unlocked the door. She loved watching the soap opera *General Hospital,* and the only TV was in our bedroom. "If the curtains were closed," Kara says, "that meant I had to go to my friend's house to watch it. I knew closed curtains signaled that Mom was depressed." Michael says he is "a little slower than the kids to recognize it." The keys for him are finding mail still in the door in the afternoon, or my begging off from dinners and meetings I normally would relish. Sandy Bakalar, a dear friend who introduced me to Michael when John and I came to Boston after the divorce, has the most poetic description. While my normal pace is nonstop, she says, when I am down "it's a slow movement. It is the slowest movement of the symphony."

My many doctors have put names to my illness that reflect their evolving perceptions of me and their profession's evolving lingo. Initially they simply called it depression, or major depression. Dr. Ned Cassem, former chief of psychiatry at Massachusetts General, noticed that the downtimes sometimes alternated with a mania in a way that suggested bipolar, but the mania was tame enough that he called me bipolar II. He also noticed that my depression generally arrived in the fall, like a despised but expected guest, persisted through the endless winter, and went away in spring. He and others termed that seasonal affective disorder or, quite aptly, SAD. Later, my therapist speculated that my spending sprees and other occasional mania were brought on by antidepressants, so he labeled my condition bipolar III. The doctors are in greater agreement about my symptoms, which range from an inability to sleep and a loss of libido to "empty nest issues."

My depression, like so many other people's, has a strong genetic link and family component. My dad had symptoms of it. So do others in my extended family, unfortunately, although theirs and his were nowhere as serious as mine. Michael, by contrast, is the most positive thinker I have ever known. That's his constitution. Yet he has been surrounded by depression throughout his life—not just mine and my family's but his brother Stelian's. He experienced his own profound self-criticism after the election loss in 1988, although he had the physical and psychological strength to built a new, positive career centered around teaching, mentoring, and advocating for everything from railroads to refugees.

My strongest family connection to depression is Mother, in more ways than just DNA. Like most people, my feelings about myself were shaped in childhood, a time when I was judged and found wanting by one of the most influential people in my life, Jane Goldberg Dickson. "You're just pretty," Mother told me when I was a little girl. "You have the looks, but your sister has the personality." What a devastating thing to say to a child! I cannot imagine making such a superficial pronouncement to any of my three children or pitting them against one another that way. My mother not only burdened me with this, she repeated it to my sister. Jinny was understandably wounded at being dubbed less attractive, and I was furious at being classified as merely pretty. How I envied Jinny for having "personality."

Mother was the most reticent person I have ever known. Attractive, refined, rigid—she was all of those. So much of what I felt about myself came from her. She died in 1977 and, for seven years after her death, I never bought a dress without wondering whether she would have approved. There was always a certain way of doing things and it was her way, even when it came to entering our home. The front door was off-limits. I remember once, in the first or second grade, making a May Day flower basket for Mother, attaching it to the front-door knob, then ringing that doorbell. She was so angry, before she saw the basket. She would be horrified about the memoir I wrote after the presidential campaign, and about this book. "Airing your laundry in public," she would have called it. Or "Kitty not knowing when to keep quiet." Dad's gregariousness and Mother's guardedness were the two poles. I was much more like my dad, much more open, but since Mother was around much more I was raised under her watchful, disapproving eye.

There are two more things you should know about Mother to know about me and my illness. The first is that she was adopted, and that I didn't find out until I was eighteen. I was a counselor at a summer camp when a cousin on my mother's side came to visit. I had a long conversation with her during which she inadvertently revealed a secret my mother had kept hidden from almost everyone, including Jinny and me. Mother was an adopted child, and the couple my sister and I called Grandfather and Grandmother actually were adoptive grandparents. When my cousin mentioned this, I was bowled over. Who could hear such a tale and not be? Soon as I got home I confronted her with what I had learned. All she said was, "Well, now you know." Then she resumed dusting the furniture. As far as she was concerned, that settled the matter. As far as I was concerned, there had been a perfidious breach of faith. I found out later that Dad knew about it and wanted to tell us, but Mother never would let him. A scant year after my mother admitted she was adopted, I started using amphetamines. Thirty-five years later, I was still sufficiently disconcerted by her answer that I chose her phrasing, "Now you know," as the title for my memoir that came out in 1990.

The last thing about Mother and me is that an addiction to diet pills wasn't the only affliction we shared. She never cooked a meal—never even puttered around the kitchen—without a glass of vermouth within reach. I'm not saying my mother was an alcoholic; truthfully, I can recall only one occasion when she had too much to drink. I am saying that based on what I have experienced and learned, Mother depended on diet pills and may have been addicted to alcohol as well. And as with me, I think Mother's dependencies grew out of a deep-seated and difficult-to-face melancholy. She had real mood swings. She got no treatment that I know of. She was a very private person who did not share that kind of information. I don't remember her ever talking about not feeling well mentally or any of that stuff. But I sensed that she had a very difficult childhood. Her relationship with her adoptive mother was always problematic. My dad alluded to, but never was definitive about, her father abusing her. Dad often said to Jinny and me that we should be understanding about Mother, given her background; we never were sure what he meant. I think part of Mother's rigidness, her perfectionism, was an attempt to keep her world from imploding and dull her psychic pain.

I now acknowledge my mother's influence as a role model, with drugs, drinking, and depression. I understand that her demands were impossible to meet, for me or anyone else. But I know that my mother helped rescue me when I got divorced nearly fifty years ago. I know that she adored Michael, pitched in any way she could with my kids and my home, and really did love me. That never should have been in doubt. She was always there for me. I also know now that while Mother had a profound effect on me, my depression along with my addictions are my responsibility—

and the only way I am going to overcome them is by taking charge rather than assigning blame.

I have told you what my illness has looked like to my family, and the role family may have played in spawning it. To complete the picture, I need to explain what that depression is like for me. I draw the shutters and retreat into myself. My energy is low, emotions all point down, contacts are difficult to sustain. Exercise becomes a chore, yet I lose weight because food no longer interests me. I tell people I am not feeling right sized, by which I mean that nothing in my mood or awareness fits my life or the world. For many who suffer from it, melancholia is a tsunami that arrives in an instant. For me it is a building backwash. I wake one morning without my usual enthusiasm for the day ahead. I can count on successive days being worse. Some people can point to a concrete cause, like a loss or illness. I have never been able to pinpoint a particular stimulus. Make that almost never. The presidential election had kept me focused, and, despite our premonitions of loss, I was relatively upbeat. After the defeat, the gloom returned and my negativism fed on itself.

People ask what the difference is between depression and sadness. Sadness has to do with some circumstance like my father's death. I listen to music at a concert or in a car and tears come to my eyes, remembering the orchestra he led and the relationship he and I had. Sadness like that is fleeting, it is not a constant. Depression is. It takes ahold of me in a very grasping way and lasts for months. When I am sad I cry. When I am depressed I don't cry. I can't.

Depression is a dark cloud that is always over me.

Four

SERENDIPITY AND SCIENCE

Death was not an option this time. A laboratory lined with jars of meticulously preserved brains was a reminder of the hundreds of dogs Professor Ugo Cerletti had sacrificed to confirm his theory that electricity could generate an epileptic attack capable of relieving the severest mental illnesses. The experiments also had made clear how to keep his subjects alive, or so Cerletti believed. Now came the ultimate test: For the first time, his patient was a person.

The hospital room where Cerletti was working with his sextet of assistants that April day in 1938 was isolated enough and the time was early enough that there was no chance of their being disturbed, but the man they called the Maestro was not satisfied. He sent a young aide into the corridors every few minutes to ensure there were no snoops. Cerletti knew the stakes. He had the ideal subject, a thirty-nine-year-old engineer from Milan brought to Rome's Clinic of Nervous and Mental Illnesses by police who found him wandering the train station without a ticket, delusional. No one claimed him as theirs or could interpret his ramblings about telepathic influences. Doctors diagnosed him as schizophrenic and offered no prospect of recovery. But Cerletti realized that, scary as his patient's condition was, the public would be even more alarmed by his proposed cure. The only other circumstance in which a subject had intentionally been infused with current was in the United States, which had designed special electric chairs to execute its most heinous criminals. The maverick professor knew he had just one chance to demonstrate that electrifying his patient's brain not only would not kill him but could be healing.

The patient, whom police referred to by the initials S.E., lay with his head at the foot of the bed, his scalp shaved, wide awake. An assistant stuck into his mouth a tube lined with gauze. A nurse used an elastic band to attach to his temples two electrodes drenched in a salt solution. At Cerletti's signal another colleague flipped a switch on the crude machine that mediated the voltage and duration of wall current dispatched to the subject's head. The timer buzzed, marking off a power surge of eighty volts lasting two-tenths of a second. S.E. shuddered, his heart racing. Falling back onto the bed, he began belting out a ribald tune, then resumed his characteristic silence.

"Someone got nervous and suggested whisperingly that the subject be allowed to rest," Cerletti recalled afterward. "Others advised a new application to be put off to the morrow. Our patient sat quietly in bed, looking about him. Then, of a sudden, hearing the low-toned conversation around him, he exclaimed—no longer in his incomprehensible jargon, but in so many clear words and in a solemn tone—'Not a second. Deadly!'"

But Cerletti persisted, ordering his assistants to ramp up the voltage to 110, the machine's maximum, and keep it on for a full half second. S.E. responded with the same spasm as before, only this time others followed, signaling a true seizure. At that point he "stopped breathing; his face was pale, then cyanotic," Dr. Ferdinando Accornero, one of Cerletti's assistants that day, recounted a half century later in a medical publication. "I listened with my stethoscope; his heart beat faster and faster."

Another colleague ticked off the time since the patient had inhaled his last breath. Five seconds. Ten. Fifteen. S.E.'s face had turned bright purple; his body was writhing. Twenty. Twenty-five. Thirty. "The heart rate kept increasing," said Accornero. "I could feel his pulse getting stronger under my fingers. 'Thirty-five . . . forty . . .' The shakes became less frequent. The muscles relaxed. 'Forty-five . . .' At the 48th second, the patient emitted a stertorous breath and became less cyanotic, and his pulse normalized. We sighed with relief."

Cerletti picks up the story: "The patient sat up of his own accord, looked about him calmly with a vague smile, as though asking what was expected of him. I asked him: 'What has been happening to you?' He answered, with no more gibberish: 'I don't know; perhaps I have been asleep.' That is how the first epileptic fit experimentally induced in man through the electric stimulus took place. So electroshock was born; for such was the name I forthwith gave it."

From then until now, S.E., the man known only by a monogram, has been a poster child for a therapy that would also be known by its initials, ECT. After ten more seizure sessions S.E. snapped out of his near-catatonia—Accornero had likened him to "a tree that does not give fruit"—and engaged with the world. Two months after his first treatment he was reunited with his wife and after that with his work. A year after his therapy he was still living at home and working at his old job. S.E. had confirmed not only that a patient could survive shock treatment but that he could thrive.

It was a eureka moment not just for Cerletti and his colleagues in Rome, but for the psychiatric specialty and medical science. Doctors back then were almost as frustrated as patients at their incapacity to cure or even control debilitating mental illnesses like schizophrenia and melancholia. They could open up the body and observe the way the heart sputtered, cancer mushroomed, and other physical ailments progressed, but what went on inside the tightly wired brain remained an enigma. Sigmund Freud had died the year before, leaving behind invaluable tools of analysis, but they were more helpful with neuroses than with the deep-seated depressions and psychoses that researchers later would learn were chemically based. The first effective psychotropic drugs were nearly a generation away. Referring to their vocation as a funereal science, psychiatrists were willing to try anything, and did, from refrigeration therapy that kept patients at ten to twenty degrees below their normal body temperature for days at a time, to tranquilizer chairs that bound to a seat their arms, wrists, and feet.

No treatment offered greater hope, or caught on more quickly, than the one Cerletti was testing that day in his laboratory. It is easy, with the controversy of subsequent eras, to forget how promising electroshock was in its earliest days. Those high expectations were reflected in the respected *Science News Letter,* which in 1940 ran its first article on shock treatment. "An electric shock, shot directly through the brain, provides new hope for bringing patients back from the living death of mental disease to mental health," the reporter gushed. "Coming at a time when war is subjecting the population of the whole world to those intolerable mental strains that precipitate mental disease, this new use of electricity for mental health instead of for death is being enthusiastically welcomed by the medical profession. . . .

"It is hoped that the day may come when the man or woman suffering from delusions, abnormal fears, split personality, or a regression into fixed posture and mutism may some day be cured simply in his own home or a local hospital by a physician who places two electrodes on the distressed head and then just plugs in on ordinary house current stepped down to the harmless voltages used."

Psychiatrists were equally ebullient. Electroshock gave them their first key to getting patients measurably better and to clearing out the back wards of state mental asylums. By the 1950s, as historian of psychiatry Edward Shorter notes, "A patient hospitalized for depression stood an excellent chance of receiving ECT, and an even better chance of benefiting from it." Dr. Max Hamilton, namesake of the most popular scale for measuring depression, went a step further, reportedly telling a colleague that "if the doctor didn't give ECT [for resistant depression], he should be charged with incompetence."

∽

The ancient Greeks were the first to dream of an electric cure. They believed there were special curative powers, even divine ones, in the seizures of epileptics. The early Romans put those powers to the test by treating head pain with help from a family of fish called Torpedinidae, or torpedo rays, which generate an electric pulse potent enough to produce a convulsion. "Headache even if it is chronic and unbearable is taken away and remedied forever by a live black torpedo placed on the spot which is in pain, until the pain ceases," Scribonius Largus, the court physician, wrote in A.D. 46. Scribonius was sufficiently confident that he tried the remedy on Emperor Claudius—the sovereign survived, although it is unclear if he was cured—then extended the treatment to ailments such as gout, and even to mental illness.

Electricity came back onto center stage in the mid-1700s. Benjamin Franklin was using kites to help unmask the mysteries of lightning. Doctors in Europe and America likewise were drawn to electricity, but for them the allure was the same as it had been for the Ancients: its power to heal. Every other year since 1744, France's Histoire de L'Académie Royal des Sciences had published a report on "Electricity and Medicine." Dispatches on supposed cures poured in from across the continent. One, in 1755, was a case of hysterical blindness in which the first thrust of current let the patient see faint rays of light, while the third had him screaming, fainting, and starting to regain full sight. Franklin also became intrigued by electricity as therapy, wiring up his subjects and trying to stun them out of paralysis and even hysteria. The results, he wrote, were arresting, albeit fleeting.

In the nineteenth century the techniques grew more sophisticated and the claims more far-reaching. The Frenchman G.B.C. Duchenne insisted in 1855 that electrotherapy was a must-do for every serious neurologist. A decade later, Rudolph Arndt, a German psychiatrist, unveiled a 130-page study on electricity's effectiveness in battling psychopathology. Such encouraging findings attracted entrepreneurs along with flimflam artists. An 1882 ad in the *Boston Globe* touted the "electrifier" as "able to cure All cases of Rheumatism, Diseases of the Liver, Stomach and Kidneys, Lung Complaints, Paralysis, Lost Vitality, Nervous Disability, Female Complaints." In 1901, the Sears, Roebuck catalog trumpeted an eighteen-dollar Giant Power Heidelberg Electric Belt, which presumably would bestow psychological as well as physical benefits by invigorating those "suffering from any trouble of the sexual organs."

Electricity, however, is just half of electroshock's bloodline. It is the stimulus that sparks a reaction. The reaction itself—the seizure or shock—is the other half, and its roots again run to Rome. Celsus the Platonist, a literary stalwart during the reign of Marcus Aurelius, used flogging and even starving to shock into balance his patients' appetites and memories. Fast forward to the sixteenth century and the renowned Swiss occultist and physician Theophrastus Bombast von Hohenheim, who gave oral doses of the crystalline compound camphor to generate convulsions that he boasted could cure lunacy. While Bombast von Hohenheim had few adherents in his era, in 1764 Dr. Leopold Auenbrugger von Auenbrugg of Vienna reported administering camphor every two hours, day and night, to treat "mania virorum." And in 1851, a Hungarian manuscript documented use of the drug to generate an epileptic attack that, once it eased, relieved a patient's mania and returned him to reason.

Despite that early promise, convulsive therapy essentially disappeared for three-quarters of a century—until the early 1900s, when there was an explosion of interest in new biological modes of treating mental illness. The first was malarial therapy, a technique made popular in Vienna in 1917 by Dr. Julius Wagner-Jauregg. For half a century scientists had been intrigued by the way psychiatric patients who contracted fever-producing diseases sometimes saw their mental health improve. Wagner-Jauregg injected blood from malaria sufferers into a series of patients with neurosyphilis, one of his era's dreaded diseases that started with sexually transmitted syphilis and often ended with dementia, paralysis, and death. The injections worked, returning his patients to near-normal lives. This so-called fever cure ultimately proved unwieldy and even dangerous and was supplanted by penicillin, but it touched off a scramble for other physical remedies for psychiatric maladies and earned Warner-Jauregg a Nobel Prize.

Sleep therapy was the next great hope. As early as 1897 a Scottish-trained physician tried sleep-inducing drugs on his manic and alcoholic patients, and it seemed to cure them. But it was Swiss psychiatrist Jakob Klaesi, himself manic-depressive, who popularized this unusual approach by treating diseases as unyielding as schizophrenia and as epidemic as depression. The technique was straightforward: give patients drugs that put them to sleep for as little as one day or as long as ten—enough time, Klaesi wrote, to "dismantle" their defenses and make them amenable to psychoanalysis and other conventional treatments. While its use eventually was constrained by its death toll—it killed one in twenty patients—it was a critical link in the progression of organic therapies.

If standard sleep could heal, what about the deep sleep of a coma? The notion of coma as cure occurred to doctors the way so many other treatments did: serendipitously. Dr. Manfred Sakel had given small doses of insulin, a newly discovered hormone, to morphine-addicted actresses and physicians in Berlin, but only to control vomiting, diarrhea, and other symptoms of withdrawal. Sometimes the insulin sent the patient into a hypoglycemic coma; when he woke he seemed more peaceful and less interested in morphine. Sakel tried intentionally inducing such comas in schizophrenics, with spectacular results. Symptoms fully cleared in thirty-five of fifty test subjects and partly remitted in another nine, he announced in 1934. The treatment quickly spread to Switzerland, Britain, and America. Thousands of patients were given increasing doses of insulin that put them to sleep, then into the deeper unconsciousness of a coma that could last for hours and occasionally was accompanied by convulsions. A solution of sugar brought them back to life—and often to a saner state—presumably having killed off diseased cells and allowing healthy ones to regenerate.

That pattern of pulling patients in and out of coma was repeated daily for up to two months. Sometimes the effects were excruciating, as they were for mathematical genius and Nobel Laureate John Nash. He fell into madness in 1960 and, when nothing else helped, he was given insulin coma treatment five days a week for six weeks. "His body would become as rigid as if it were frozen solid and his fingers would be curled," Nash's biographer, Sylvia Nasar, wrote in *A Beautiful Mind*. "At that point, a nurse would put a rubber hose through his nose and esophagus, and a glucose solution would be administered. . . . Then he would wake up, slowly and agonizingly. . . . Very often, during the comatose stage, patients whose blood-sugar levels dropped too far would have spontaneous seizures—thrashing around, biting their tongues. Broken bones were not uncommon. Sometimes patients remained in the coma." Nash later acknowledged that the treatments, monstrous though they seemed, were the beginning of his getting better. And in those early days in the 1930s, it was only Sakel's successes that were trumpeted, such as when he freed ballet master Vaslav Nijinsky from the Swiss sanatorium where he had been confined.

"Is it any wonder that asylum psychiatrists became keen about insulin coma?" asks historian Edward Shorter. "It seemed to be a procedure that actually worked, at least for the short term, without the extreme dangerousness of sleep therapy. In the long term, it was discovered that insulin coma had about the same success rate as barbiturate-sleep therapy. Both represented a substantial improvement on what was available before, which is to say, nothing."

At the same time that Sakel was exploring the mysterious properties of insulin, Hungarian doctor Ladislas von Meduna was mesmerized by the seeming antagonism between schizophrenia and epilepsy. Postmortem examination of the brains of epileptic patients revealed a profusion of the delicate network of branched cells that support and protect nerves, while brains of schizophrenic patients had hardly any. That difference assumed practical significance when a colleague pointed out that the onset of schizophrenia in epileptics seemed to cure them of their epilepsy. Meduna wondered whether the reverse might be true: Could epileptic-like seizures relieve schizophrenia? His challenge back in 1933, as he later recounted, was "to find a convulsant drug which could be used safely in human beings, which would produce epileptic attacks by acting upon the nerve cells of the brain, and which would leave the cerebral blood vessels intact."

Meduna ran through a series of potions, from strychnine to caffeine, eventually settling on a milder version of the camphor compound that von Hohenheim had tried four hundred years earlier. After proving it safe with guinea pigs, Meduna did his first human experiment on January 23, 1934. His subject, known only as L. Zoltan, was a thirty-three-year-old schizophrenic who for four years had been in a catatonic stupor. He heard voices emanating from his stomach and was unable to move or eat on his own. Meduna injected an oily camphor solution into Zoltan's right buttock, then nervously stepped back. "After 45 minutes of anxious and fearful waiting," Meduna wrote fifty years afterward, "the patient suddenly had a classical epileptic attack that lasted 60 seconds. During the period of observation I was able to maintain my composure . . . but when the attack was over and the patient recovered his consciousness, my legs suddenly gave out. My body began to tremble, a profuse sweat drenched me, and, as I later heard, my face was ashen gray." While Meduna was relieved, Zoltan was not. Not yet. He survived his grand mal seizure, but it took five injections and five convulsions until, on February 10, "for the first time in four years, [Zoltan] got out of his bed, began to talk, requested breakfast, dressed himself without help, was interested in everything around him, and asked about his disease, and how long he had been in the hospital. When we told him that he spent four years at the hospital he did not believe it. He looked like Rip Van Winkle who spent years in sleep, and gained a better and better orientation from minute to minute."

After several more ups and down, Zoltan one night escaped from the hospital, headed home, and, as the head nurse later recounted to Meduna, Zoltan "found out that the cousin living with his wife was not a relation at all but his wife's lover. He beat up the cousin and kicked him out of the house; proceeded to beat up his wife and told her that he is not going to live in a crazy world where things like that could happen, and that he prefers to live in the state mental hospital where there is peace and honesty, and he came back." From then on, Meduna added, "I considered this patient cured, and he remained well at the time I left Europe in 1939."

Zoltan was not an aberration. Meduna published results showing that 10 out of 26 schizophrenic patients completely recovered. Camphor was soon replaced with a synthetic cardiac stimulant called Cardiazol, or Metrazol as it was known in the United States, which worked even faster. Again, Meduna's results were encouraging: 41 out of 110 patients totally remitted.

Whereas convulsions were neither necessary for nor a key element of what Sakel had in mind with his insulin coma treatment, they were the central therapeutic ingredient with Metrazol. Yet the two new treatments had a lot in common. Both signaled the arrival of the biological era in psychiatry. Both relied on jolting the brain into an agitated state, hence their being lumped together by historians as the first shock therapies. And, like insulin coma, Metrazol spread too quickly, outpacing a rigorous analysis of its benefits and a realistic weighing of its risks. Doctors were unable to control the intensity of Metrazol-induced convulsions, which led to patients suffering broken bones, ripped muscles, and teeth pried loose. "Just before the convulsion one patient said: 'I am sorry, I am dying—Forgive me . . . [another] patient was sure that embalming fluid was injected into his veins," Washington-based psychiatrist

Solomon Katzenelbogen reported in 1940, at a time when Metrazol was being used to treat everything from schizophrenia to depression, mania, and alcoholism. "While the patients' statements obviously reflect some of the content of their basic psychotic conditions, they contain nevertheless one common and outstanding feature, namely, the feeling of being tortured, and of intense fear of imminent death."

Other side effects included erections, ejaculation, and involuntary urination and defecation, wrote Katzenelbogen, whose article today reads like an unofficial obituary for the procedure. The problem was not the treatment itself, which had an impressive track record, but "that this very drastic procedure is becoming routine practice. Instead of being reserved for special, particularly ominous conditions, it is being used rather indiscriminately, without due regard for the nature and seriousness of the illness."

⌒

Maestro Cerletti never set out to tame mental illness. While Sakel and Meduna fantasized about relieving or even resolving the severest mental maladies, Cerletti's aim in 1933 was more modest and practical: to unravel the thickening he had observed in the brains of epileptics. Was the lesion the *cause* of their epilepsy, or, as he suspected, was it a *consequence* of the repeated convulsions they had endured?

To find the answer, Cerletti needed to induce a convulsion in his test animals—without altering their brain in a way that would mask whether the effect was caused by the convulsion itself or by the induction agent. Drugs were too diffuse. Electricity was targeted enough, but Cerletti worried that repeatedly passing a current directly through the brain would produce the same uncontrolled cell changes as drugs. A colleague suggested an alternative approach: apply one electrode in the animal's mouth, the other in the rectum, to spare the brain while still sparking a seizure. Cerletti already had decided on dogs as the most easily available, anatomically appropriate animal to test, and he tried the oral-anal electric approach on scores of them at his laboratory in Genoa. The hounds experienced precisely the convulsions the researchers were seeking. It was not a pretty process. The dogs bit their tongues even as urine and feces flowed uncontrollably from their bottoms. At first most of the animals died, but by applying less current Cerletti and his assistants were able to induce the seizure *and* keep the animals alive, at least until he decided to dissect their brains.

Intent as he was on his research, Cerletti had a mind too active and a soul too fiery to stay narrowly focused on epileptic lesions. And too much was happening around him for the brilliant young physician not to be seduced away from the laboratory. Psychiatry was being revitalized, with a new sense of its power to heal, just as he was being summoned to chair the Department of Neuropsychiatry at the University of Rome's medical college. Then there was Sakel's work on insulin coma, which Cerletti was schooled in by the founder himself. Meduna, meanwhile, had scored his breakthrough with Cardiazol convulsions, and Cerletti quickly introduced the therapy to his clinic. Coma and Cardiazol made clear to Cerletti that convulsions could be healing rather than just harmful, and made the Maestro wonder whether electricity might offer a more benign way to treat the mentally ill than a harsh drug like Cardiazol. "This possibility we often discussed at our Institute," he wrote looking back, "and particularly when observing, after cardiazol injections, the painful reactions which shook fully conscious patients for over a minute—as a result most of them refused the subsequent treatments."

So, in the fall of 1936, Cerletti dispatched his assistants to the pressing questions that begged answering. One would school himself in the ways Cardiazol worked. A second, Accornero, was to become an expert in insulin therapy. Dr. Lucio Bini, considered the coinventor of ECT, was given the momentous task of designing a shock device fine-tuned enough to induce a convulsion in humans without harming them.

Bini and Cerletti tested their theories not just on dogs, but on pigs at the slaughterhouse in Rome. Butchers used electricity to stun and convulse the animals, making it easier to kill and bleed them. The slaughterhouse experience proved two critical things: that current could be applied directly to the head and that the dose of electricity needed to provoke a seizure would not be life threatening to a hog or, presumably, to a human. His experiments on pigs "caused all my doubts to vanish," the Maestro explained. "Without more ado I gave instructions in the clinic to undertake, next day, the experiment upon man."

That man was S.E., the schizophrenic engineer from Milan, and his recovery made Cerletti and his team rightfully feel as if they were at the edge of something momentous. One patient followed another, as the Rome researchers sought to generate findings on efficacy and safety that could be generalized to a wider population. "We agreed to have each session announced with the sound of a trumpet to gather all the physicians in the clinic who might be interested in the event. For an entire year the aide, Spartaco, played an out-of-tune trumpet three or four times a week," Accornero wrote. "After about 1 year of work, the results of our studies were published, and any physician was then able to use electroshock with an adequate technique."

All that was left was to put a name to the new procedure. One assistant suggested electric shock; Cerletti objected because it was already used for muscle contractions directly due to electricity. Ditto for electro-convulsion. Another aide proposed electroshake, which Cerletti thought too scary. So he ended with electroshock, a moniker that today is used more by the therapy's critics than its supporters, and that its inventor himself later said he regretted. Cerletti, meanwhile, was telling friends that the novel therapy was not an invention, merely an audacious act.

⧼⧽

Electroshock's invention may or may not have been audacious, but the speed of its spread certainly was. That was partly a function of the deficiencies with earlier biological treatments, especially Metrazol, the dominant psychiatric procedure of the day. Electric shock was simpler to apply, with none of Metrazol's difficulty finding a vein through which to infuse it. Electric convulsions were shorter, less violent, and less dreaded by patients, partly because they blacked out during electroshock but remained wide awake with Metrazol. There was also less chance of extra and unintended seizures when electricity was used, and it was less likely to break bones, aggravate other medical conditions, or kill the patient. Add to that its relatively low cost and short treatment time, and electroshock quickly trumped drugs as the preferred method to induce a seizure.

Even more critical to understanding the popularity of all the convulsive treatments is appreciating how little else there was back then, and how much of that was gimmickry if not quackery. The eugenics movement that was sweeping across America and eventually was picked up by Hitler and his Aryan henchmen was fueled by the notion that the mentally ill were unfit to reproduce. Over the first half of the twentieth century eugenicists in the United States sterilized more than twenty thousand patients in state mental hospitals. Another popular asylum cure was "hydrotherapy," where patients were strapped for hours or even days onto a hammock hung inside a bathtub, then drenched in alternating cold and hot water, all with the aim of exhausting them physically and reviving them mentally. If changing their nurture did not work, why not change their very nature? Sometimes it was the uterus or ovaries that were surgically removed, other times an entire row of teeth or several feet of bowel, the goal in each case being to rid the body of an organ said to be poisoning the mind.

Treatments like those earned mental hospitals their reputation as snake pits. The desperation that led psychiatrists to latch on to cockeyed therapies coincided with and was fueled by a surge in population that, in America, saw the number of mental patients more than double from 143,000 in 1903 to 366,000 in 1933. Most were categorized under the catchall of schizophrenia, although they suffered a range of disabling and seemingly incurable conditions. "Today's psychiatrists do not realize that those of us working in psychiatric hospitals before the 1930s could do little more for our patients than make them comfortable, maintain contact with their families, and in case of a spontaneous remission, return them to the community," Dr. Lothar Kalinowsky recalled half a century later.

Electroshock could not cure those warehoused patients, but it relieved their symptoms and suffering enough that it spread across Europe, then to the United States and other far-flung lands. Kalinowsky, a German-Jewish psychiatrist who had fled Hitler in 1933, played such a central role in that transmission that he came to be called the Johnny Appleseed of ECT. He was in Rome in the early days with Cerletti, then brought the new therapy to Paris in 1939. That summer, he and electroshock arrived in England, again taking haven from the Nazis and again planting the therapy in new soil. In 1940, the itinerant professor landed in America, and that fall he helped launch one of this country's first and most storied electroshock programs at Columbia University and the affiliated New York Psychiatric Institute.

By the time Kalinowsky treated his first patient in September 1940, another patient had already been treated in New York earlier that year, and ECT programs had been or soon would be established in university or private clinics in Philadelphia, Boston, Chicago, Washington, and Cincinnati. In short order, however, the bulk of treatments were being given in public mental asylums, which housed the bulk of the sickest patients. A 1945 article gives a flavor of those treatments at Rochester State Hospital, which had administered 5,000 shock sessions to 350 patients and was doing 100 new ones a week. Doctors were shocking so many patients that they needed what amounted to an assembly line, the author wrote, where "while one patient is being treated in the shock room, another is being adjusted on the second table and can then be wheeled in as soon as the first patient leaves the room. Thus a continuous stream of patients is maintained and by this method 30 patients can be treated in about one and one-half hours."

Four out of every ten patients at Rochester and other hospitals of that era suffered a serious complication—a rate four hundred times higher than today—with most involving dislocations or fractures. That is not surprising since patients were wide awake at the start of the procedure and doctors were using a rudimentary muscle relaxant or none at all. The jaw was a special problem, with patients clenching hard enough to make their gums bleed. Sprains and breaks were also common in the neck, spine, shoulder, and even the head. To minimize the risk, "the patient's arms are pinioned at his sides by means of a folded sheet which envelops the chest and abdomen. A wide canvas strap restrains the knees. . . . Shoes are always worn to guard against fractures of the [heel bone]. Manual restraint is performed in the customary way by an attendant on each side. . . . A padded tongue depressor is placed between the teeth."

Those early patients often let out a shriek as the electricity was applied, but as they convulsed they blacked out. Medical precautions were taken to guard against the same dangers that worry ECT doctors today, but back then they were rudimentary. A sufficient flow of oxygen was ensured not with today's respirators but by urging the patient "to take several deep breaths." A similar approach was taken to restore a patient's airway after the convulsion: "The operator then straightens the trachea by placing a hand behind the neck and holding the head in extended position by a firm grip on the hair with the other hand." Or, more simply, "blowing against the face." As for dislocations of the jaw, they were tended to after the fact "by placing the thumb inside the mouth at the angle of the jaw and reducing the dislocation by means of downward and backward pressure."

Depressed patients generally needed ten treatments at Rochester State. Those with progressive paranoia got fifteen. Twenty or more were needed for "schizoid types."

Other hospitals found it more efficient to have patients stay where they were and bring the machine to them. "Patients were lined up in a large dormitory and treated en masse," recalls Dr. Zigmond Lebensohn, himself an ECT pioneer. "With their heads at the foot of the bed, the ECT apparatus was wheeled from patient to patient, accompanied by the doctor and his assistants. This permitted a large number of treatments to be administered in a very short period." Some treatments were given in doctors' offices. In rare cases, Lebensohn writes, "the psychiatrist would make a 'house call' with his ECT machine, accompanied by a nurse or an assistant, and the treatment would be administered in the patient's own bed. Responsible members of the patient's family were instructed to remain with the patient until recovery was complete."

The focus was less on electroshock's process and more on its pain for anyone lying on the shock bed looking up, the way thousands of patients were. "A counterpane was pulled up to my neck and a small straw pillow, though covered with a clean towel, was wet with the sweat of the men who had gone before," said a twenty-four-year-old chemist whose account of his electroshock treatment for manic depression was published anonymously by his doctor in 1948. "I was wheeled out into the hall to wait my turn. There was another scream and a gurgling coughing groan, and the patient ahead of me was moved out down the hall and into the dormitory, with arms and legs and head flopping around. Before I realized it I was zooming down the hall. . . . I was mighty scared and there was no use kidding about it. Mac [an attendant and former patient] held my right arm and pressed hard with the elbow just inside my shoulder muscle. Sarge [a hospital staffer] had the other arm. Another attendant climbed up on the wagon and lay across my knees gripping the side of the wagon with hands and toes. The three attendants would hold me down during my convulsion. [Some hospitals referred to this technique as "riding the patient."] The theory was: The more severe the convulsion, the better the results.

"I heard the doctor give the pretty blonde nurse a set of numbers, and I knew that she was setting the dials. 'God, don't let her give me an overdose.' Mac's face was about eight inches above my own. I looked up into Mac's eyes. Mac wasn't smiling a bit. I stared up into Mac's eyes and slowly said over and over to myself, 'Mac, you big Irish lug, take care of me now.' Very deliberately, very slowly a black shade came up over my eyes."

If his apprehension was understandable, his relief afterward was a surprise. "I woke up sometime later feeling completely refreshed, not tired or logy, or drugged with sleep, just ready for a big day," the young patient recounted. "What had the shock treatment done for me? It had given me a new chance. I was able to start over fresh. With no memory, no delusions, no fears. Or at least I had no memory of them for that period of days before I could again remember the details of my life. In that time I had been reoriented. I was on the right track for the first time in some years."

Electroshock was trying for that patient as for most others, but it was the only treatment that gave them the chance to get better, and word about it was getting out. Just how fast shock was catching on became clear in a U.S. Public Health Service survey in October 1941, barely eighteen months after the treatment arrived in America. While nearly four times as many patients were getting the older insulin coma therapy, and five times as many got Metrazol, the future was all electroshock. Two-thirds of hospitals responded that they were stepping up their use of electrically induced seizures, while only 10 and 14 percent were doing more insulin and Metrazol, respectively. Fully one-third had discontinued insulin and Metrazol treatments, while only one of the 129 hospitals offering electroshock had canceled the program.

McLean Hospital, in the Boston suburb of Belmont, was part of that trend. In a 1942 report to the Public Health Service, the hospital's director explained that McLean had stopped using insulin shock in 1939 because of the "risk of brain damage, unimpressive therapeutic results, impracticality of the elaborate needs of the therapeutic management." It stopped using Metrazol in 1941 because of "preference of electrical stimulation, because of greater precision in control of application . . . apparently also less risk of brain damage."

Psychiatrists on the Pacific Coast were even more ebullient. At Stockton State Hospital, California's first insane asylum, doctors got their first ECT machine in 1943. That year they treated 52 patients; by 1948 the count was up to 604. The following year new machines were purchased, enough to treat 2,997 patients. "Underscoring its status as the 'foremost method of therapy in the state hospitals,' doctors shocked 60 percent of the patients at Stockton that year," reports Dr. Joel Braslow, a historian who conducted a study of Stockton.

By the end of the 1940s, insulin, electric shock, or both were being used in "about nine-tenths of the mental hospitals in the country," the *New York Times* reported in April 1949. Most of the rest would, too, if they had the money and staff, the paper concluded based on a national survey. The majority of the 370 hospitals polled said they preferred insulin to treat schizophrenia, although because of its high cost many were using electroshock instead. Electrically induced seizures were the favored treatment for depression. No mention was made of Metrazol, presumably because it no longer was a factor. A *Times* story the following month said that in a study of one hundred schizophrenic patients at a New York hospital, electric shock "produced results twice as successful as under earlier systems of treatment."

Schizophrenia and depression were the primary ailments where shock was prescribed, but far from the only ones. It was tried with alcoholism, morphine addiction, ulcerative colitis, and even homosexuality. A pair of doctors from Columbia University presented one such case in 1944, of a "21-year-old lad of highly neurotic stock" who "was a paranoid homosexual, though no overt homosexuality had been practiced except mutual masturbation in early childhood." After ten shock treatments, the doctors wrote, "he had several successful relationships with other girls, though the emotional side of his sex experience was still not completely normal. He looked more virile and stopped stammering in his hours with the analyst, a symptom of his fear of castration which had previously been outstanding and constant."*

---

*ECT doctors were not the only ones in that era trying to "cure" homosexuality. Psychiatry generally saw it as a disease, and tried treating it with everything from Freudian analysis to aversion therapy. It took until the mid-1970s for the American Psychiatric Association to remove homosexuality from its list of illnesses.

At Stockton State Hospital, Braslow found that "diagnosis mattered little in doctors' decisions to shock a patient. Electroshock proved too useful for doctors to worry themselves about a patient's diagnosis." One Stockton superintendent, who was later promoted to run the entire California mental health network, ticked off illnesses where he thought electroshock could help: "1. Depressions 2. Depressions with agitation 3. Excitements, including excitements with symptoms of exhaustion, where electric shock therapy is considered an emergency 4. Catatonic reactions 5. Paranoid reactions 6. Hebephrenics* whose illness has been of comparatively short duration." That expansive enumeration, as Braslow notes, conveyed the unmistakable message that "electroshock therapy works best on *all* psychiatric patients."

It was not just America and Europe that were embracing shock treatment. It reached India by the 1940s and was widely used there by the end of that decade. It got to Japan even earlier, just as it was arriving in the United States. It even worked its way under the Iron Curtain, although the Soviets allegedly used it for torture as well as therapy.

∞

Shock doctors were not content with the treatment they inherited. It was too prone to rattling bones and shattering teeth to attract patients, reassure families, or craft a positive public image of an unsettling-sounding treatment called electroshock.

By the time the treatment arrived in America, physicians were already experimenting with drugs to relax the muscles and reduce fractures and dislocations. Their first choice, curare, was an unfortunate one. It was made by stirring toxic bark scrapings with fragments of plants, snake venom, and even venomous ants, then boiling the witches' brew

---

*A type of schizophrenia, usually starting at puberty, characterized by delusions and hallucinations.

for two days and evaporating out a thick, bitter paste. The traditional way to test its potency was to count how many—or, more precisely, how few—leaps a frog could manage after being pricked. Alkaloids made from the mixture were already being used by doctors to relax limbs. Omaha psychiatrist Abram Bennett had tried it on children with spastic paralysis and reasoned that it should work just as well with his patients whose bones were snapping under the strain of Metrazol shock. He made an arrangement to get a big supply from Ecuador, then had it processed at the University of Nebraska's drug laboratory.

It did control thrashing, starting in 1940 with Metrazol and soon after with electroshock, but it sometimes caused what Kalinowsky termed "unpleasant incidents." What he had in mind, he explained, is "respiratory embarrassment" that "is not infrequent." It also had an effect on the heart that "is sometimes serious." What all that added up to, he said, is that "an unduly large percentage of the fatalities reported in ECT" occur in patients treated with curare.

Some doctors chose to use curare anyway, accepting the risks of side effects in return for the clear-cut benefits of reduced fractures. Most waited until a safer alternative was available, which took until 1951. Succinylcholine had been used since 1949 for easing the insertion of tracheal tubes, but it took another two years for it to catch on with shock treatments. Like curare, it went to work fast and relaxed muscles enough to eliminate most fractures of the spine and other joints; unlike the South American elixir, it was quickly expelled from the body and was largely risk-free.*

Relaxing the muscles was one big thing. Resting the mind was at least as important, and became more so with the added distress of the lungs going limp thanks to the muscle relaxant. Anesthetics—generally

---

*Curare is used in some ECT treatments today to prevent muscle soreness, but its preparation is carefully controlled in laboratories, and positive-pressure ventilation prevents the cardiac arrests of the past.

quick-acting barbiturates like Amytal or Pentothal—were introduced to electroshock in 1945 and were common by the early 1950s. More critical was ensuring the brain got enough oxygen. At the beginning it was common for ECT patients to actually stop breathing for several minutes, causing oxygen levels to plummet in their blood and brain, turning them blue, and leading to long-lasting loss of memory. By the mid-1950s, patients were getting high doses of oxygen along with their anesthesia and muscle relaxant.

That triplet of anesthesia, muscle relaxant, and oxygen transformed electroshock at least as much as Novocain remade dentistry, ridding the procedure not just of pain and injury but of many of its most frightening images. During World War II, the U.S. military trained its doctors in various psychiatric techniques, including convulsive ones, and they brought home a belief in the treatment and a knowledge of how to use it. The war also created thousands of subjects for electroshock in ex-soldiers whose suffering from combat fatigue and other stress disorders lingered long after the battles.

There were signs in those early days of the issues that would nearly kill the treatment twenty years later and continue to shadow it today. Studies documented lesions and other effects in the brain, but most researchers agreed with Louis Lowinger and James H. Huddleson of the Veterans Facility on Long Island who, in a 1946 review in the *American Journal of Psychiatry,* concluded that the changes generally are "reversible" and that EEG disturbances "tend to disappear in several months." There was also a sense, voiced in 1959 by none other than the Maestro, that the electroshock he had founded was "unesthetic—ugly." He and others were confident they could reform it, although few shared Cerletti's vision of injecting depressed patients with a solution made from the brains of hogs that had been shocked.

Early practitioners noted the memory loss experienced by many electroshock patients. But rather than fretting over or downplaying it the way doctors would over subsequent generations, shock pioneers saw it as a risk worth taking and, more important, one that could be reduced. Every one of today's techniques for doing that—from delivering current to just one side of the head rather than both, to altering the length and form of the pulse—was discussed as long ago as the 1940s. The problem was that in that "pre-science" period, ECT researchers did not have controlled trials and other rigorous experiments that would let them test their theories. Instead, psychiatrists followed the approach that was the standard then in medicine: watch how ECT was done as an intern or resident, do it the same way when you opened a practice, then teach that technique to the next generation of students.

ECT trailblazers also looked at memory loss, at least the temporary variety, as a potential key to the treatment's success. ECT works by "aiding the patients to forget their emotional problems temporarily and thus eventually breaking up the psychopathic pattern," Columbia professor of psychiatry Nolan D.C. Lewis concluded in a 1942 talk before the New York Academy of Medicine. His explanation reflected psychiatry's inclination then to see electroshock in the context of the prevailing paradigm of psychoanalysis: "In the successful case the patient has gained a more complete control over the dominating psychopathologic ideas, and the immediately favorable results are startling, even miraculous at times."

The word "miracle" was used a lot back then, by doctors, patients, and even the press. Dr. Zigmond Lebensohn was part of that era of ebullience, and recalls what it was like: "The first time I witnessed an electroconvulsive treatment in 1939, I had some of the same visceral reaction I experienced as a medical student witnessing my first surgical operation." Dr. Abraham Myerson of the Boston Psychopathic Hospital agreed. Electroshock, Myerson told his colleagues at an American Psychiatric Association meeting a few years after the treatment arrived in America, has generated "a high percentage of immediately apparent improvement unparalleled in the history of psychiatry. . . . The defeatism of former days has disappeared for many workers in the field of psychiatry, and optimism in the treatment of the mental diseases for the first time has a valid basis."

It was partly that electroshock really did work—an estimated 80 percent of patients got better. Rates of death and complications fell far and fast enough that shock displaced sleep therapy, insulin coma, Metrazol, and all the other biological treatments that had helped spawn it. Electroshock's golden age also had a lot to do with the fact that the era of psychopharmaceuticals had yet to dawn. Chlorpromazine, the antipsychotic that kicked off the revolution in drug therapy, was not approved by the U.S. Food and Drug Administration until 1954. ECT had defects, but they were not enough to derail it, not yet. For nearly two full decades after Ugo Cerletti and his team christened the electric treatment, it was the dominant technique in psychiatry and the preferred option for most psychiatrists.

Five

A LITANY OF TREATMENTS,
A DEARTH OF CURES

Every addict has her melting point. It is the stage where one more drink, or pill, can push her into oblivion. I was about to reach mine, with potentially lethal consequences, when my brother-in-law showed me a way to turn down the temperature.

I remember the date: June 20, 1982. Michael and I had been married on that day nineteen years earlier. Our wedding was a watershed event for both of us, but especially for me. It set my life on a new and optimistic course after a miserable first marriage. Michael and I have our differences, to be sure. He is frugal to the point of buying at Costco ten times what we need of everything from aspirin to breakfast cereal, then letting everyone in earshot know how much he saved. I relish Whole Foods, flying business class, and buying nice clothes, although I have learned to cut off the price tags before showing them to him. Michael takes public transit, picks up trash while walking to work, and never cashed in on the perks of public office. I prefer taxis and don't mind using my limited clout. Michael is proud of his Greek roots; I am proud of my Jewish roots. Far more unites than divides us, however, from our love of our three kids to our passions for justice and for each other. It was that devotion that kept me by his side through endless grueling campaigns. It kept him by mine through two decades of amphetamines and alcohol.

Anniversaries are a time when we remind each other of all that is magical in our marriage—and, too often, when I test his patience with yet another crisis. Number nineteen was a dramatic case in point. We had just finished an exquisite dinner at the Blue Strawbery restaurant in the old navy town of Portsmouth, where New Hampshire meets Maine. We were driving back to Boston with our dinner companions, my sister Jinny and her husband Al Peters. Al is a recovering alcoholic, now twenty-six years sober, and has always been candid about his drinking problems and bids to help other alcoholics.

"I need help," I said as we sped along the interstate. For the first time I spelled out to Al my pill-popping habit of a quarter century. I had been especially tense recently, I told him, snapping at Michael, losing my cool at Kara's grammar school graduation, and dreading another bare-knuckles campaign for governor. Michael was determined to take back the office that Ed King had wrested from him four years earlier when, as one of King's henchmen confessed to the press, "we put all the hate groups in one big pot and let it boil." To win the rematch, Michael needed to prove he was not the aloof and austere elitist King had painted him in the first go-around. And he needed my help, or at least the assurance I would not be a liability. In order to do that *I* needed help, and I felt sure Al would know where to get it.

I was right. "Addiction is addiction," Al advised. "It doesn't matter whether you take your drug in pill form, alcohol form, shoot it up, or smoke it." He sent me to a physician friend of his, who put me in touch with a woman in New York who had survived addictions to amphetamines and alcohol. I flew there to meet with her, poured out my whole sorry story, then took down information on what she said was a first-rate treatment center in Center City, Minnesota. I telephoned the clinic, called Hazelden, over the July 4 weekend. July 4 is a big deal in Boston and bigger still in my family. Our fair city rightly considers itself the birthplace of the American Revolution. To celebrate, my dad and the Boston Pops performed a nationally broadcast concert every July 4 from the banks of the Charles River. Independence Day seemed like the right moment for me to declare my independence from this ruinous drug habit, or at least to try.

When you are living in a family as political as mine, in the middle of what proved to be Michael's hardest-fought campaign for governor, checking in to a drug clinic is no small matter. Drugs were a hot-button issue then, even more than today, and addiction was almost as electrifying a political topic as mental health. Our solution was subterfuge. My health, mental or otherwise, was no one's business. We concocted a cover story in case anyone wondered why I was heading to the Midwest: I had hepatitis and was on my way to recuperate at the home of a college roommate, Anne Forgy. Hopefully no one would try to talk to my doctors, or uncover the fact that Anne lived in Missouri while my ticket was for Minnesota. My kids were in on the ruse, but not wild about lying. Michael dropped me off at Logan Airport. I wouldn't let him come in for fear someone would recognize him and start asking questions. I made it to the boarding area without seeing anyone I knew, but once there I spotted an acquaintance putting his daughters on the plane. I hid behind my book, then practically ran to my seat and kept that book in front of my face the whole flight.

A number of good things happened at Hazelden, starting with

ending my tortured romance with diet pills. The clinic's detoxification doctrine is time-tested and hard-edged. No sooner did I arrive than staffers searched my bags, opening every tube and jar, checking every pocket and suitcase lining, to make sure I was not bringing in diet pills or any other banned substance. I was assigned to a unit with twenty-four other women, given homework, and scheduled for group meetings. At midnight that first night, I was instructed to swallow four tablets of Librium, a benzodiazepine used to treat anxiety and withdrawal. It is difficult to remember much more from those first few days. The Librium and other medications barely let me stay awake. But in the end it worked. Thanks to the antidrug drugs, talk therapy, and all the rungs of Hazelden's twelve-step program, I had taken my last diet pill. I felt safe at the treatment center, freed not just from popping pills but from worrying someone would catch me sneaking them. Twenty-six years later, I finally could proclaim myself a recovering drug addict, even if I couldn't proclaim it to anyone outside my immediate family and a very few close and discreet friends.

Hazelden had a lasting and positive effect on my kids, too. Kara, Andrea, and John flew out for family support sessions, which meant living in dormitories and doing the hard work of group therapy with total strangers. It was not something a mother wants to ask of her children. Teenage summers should be spent frolicking at camp, or rollicking at the beach or in the Berkshires. Holding their drug-addicted mother's hand was not part of the kids' plan, or mine. But having to pull together for me, repeatedly, is one reason they are so very, very close today. Andrea, my daughter who is a journalist with NPR, puts it this way: "When Mom is feeling good, she is the glue that keeps the family together and having fun. When she is sad, that is the glue that unites us."

Two long-festering sores came to the surface at Hazelden. It was there I was made to face the fact that I was an alcohol addict.

I did not believe it. I had a battery of defenses. Jews were not drunks. Drunks were the kind of people we passed in the gutters, the kind I had tried to help through years of work with the homeless, not my kind. I could stop drinking anytime I wanted. I drank in small doses. I knew addiction, I had admitted mine to diet pills, but I was not addicted to wine. Or gin. Or even vodka. I agreed at Hazelden to attend meetings back in Boston of an alcohol support group, and I kept my promise—for about five months. When it came time to introduce myself at those group sessions, I freely fessed up that "I'm Kitty and I am a drug addict." But I could not bring myself to repeat what they made me say in Minnesota: that I was an alcoholic, too.

My month at Hazelden also helped me see, for the first time, that I was clinically depressed—as if drugs and alcohol weren't enough. Depression is something no one wants, but it was easier for me to accept than alcoholism. My earliest symptoms, which I felt from the moment they made me stop the diet pills, were exhaustion and depletion. I had no energy, no interest in what was going on around me, which became characteristic of later bouts of despair. There was a rabbi at Hazelden who was also a therapist. He was the first therapist I had ever seen. He said, "What you are feeling is depression." I said, "I've never been depressed before." He said, "Now you are."

Looking back, I can see that I was not deep-down depressed back then. I began feeling better after being off the diet pills for a while. I was getting therapy and facing my demons. The doctors at Hazelden put me on my first antidepressant, and it seemed to be working. I was heading back to Boston, and the last month of Michael's primary campaign, fully confident that he would win his rematch against Ed King and that I would beat back this incipient depression. I was half-right.

Michael won the election. My depression, meanwhile, looks

like it will be a lifelong curse. I almost certainly had it for years before I first acknowledged it at Hazelden, and my dreams of it vanishing with the subtraction of diet pills and the addition of antidepressants were just that, a fantasy. So were my denials. I had come a long way since that anniversary dinner in 1982 at the Blue Strawbery, facing, attacking, and defeating my drug habit. I would eventually become so comfortable with that part of my addiction history that I went public with it, although that took another five years. The day after Independence Day in 1987, I called a press conference where I told the world, or least anyone who cared, that I was a drug addict. I revealed the time I had spent at Hazelden in 1982, and boasted that I had been drug-free all that time.

Confidently fielding reporters' questions that day, I never imagined I would have to check back into Hazelden and a series of other treatment centers. My next, and the one that probably did the most good, was Edgehill Newport. Nestled on sixty-five acres in scenic Newport, Rhode Island, with a swimming pool, gym, and other amenities, it looked like an expensive resort. It was expensive, but my month there was hardly a vacation. The facility was recommended to me by Al Peters, my addiction guru, who had worked there as part of his training to become a social worker and knew how effective a rigorous, highly structured program could be. He also knew how desperate I was in February 1989. His wife, my sister Jinny, had rescued me more than once from a drink-until-I-pass-out binge. I had sunk so low that I actually had turned on John, my firstborn, telling him to mind his own goddamned business when he tried to stop me from raiding our liquor cabinet.

At Edgehill, alcohol was verboten, even in negligible quantities, which is why they confiscated my breath spray. Suicide was another worry, so they took away my razor and everyone else's. No problem with boredom, however, or wondering what to do with your day. Every minute was prescribed. We were awakened by a fellow resident, dubbed the Town Crier, who rapped on our door at 6:15 a.m. I started my day by crashing the exercise class held for cocaine addicts. Then it was breakfast in the cafeteria and a "therapeutic task." Mine was checking rooms, for which I earned the nickname Bed Ripper. I was supposed to rip apart the bed of anyone who had failed to make it. Mornings consisted of an hour of peer evaluation, then a ninety-minute meeting of our alcohol support group. After lunch I would take a walk, then go to group therapy. I found time in the afternoon for an aerobics workout, then a much-needed nap. Evenings were full, too, with films, lectures, and a story from a fellow resident.

Like all the rehab centers, Edgehill went to great lengths to protect the privacy of its patients. It went to even greater lengths with me, including letting me into a staffer's office to call Michael in the evening rather than using the more public phone. But it was in vain. Massachusetts was too nearby, too many Edgehill residents were from there, and I had by then become a national figure thanks to Michael's recently concluded presidential campaign. If people didn't recognize me by sight, they did once my name was mentioned. My first day there, five minutes after I checked in, someone dropped a dime to the *Boston Globe*. The next day Michael called a press conference to make public my drinking problems and my entering the treatment program. A day later it was national news, and reporters started hanging out around the edges of Edgehill. We had to start closing the drapes. The press simply doesn't recognize that parts of your life are private. The presence of journalists was especially unnerving when Dad, Michael, and the kids came for counseling sessions. *USA Today* took the invasion a giant step further by encouraging readers to send me get-well cards. *Newsweek* dug up teary-eyed photographs from the campaign for a pair of stories called "Roots of Addiction" and "She Clearly Recognizes She Has a Sickness." And the *Globe* ran a series of stories, including one entitled "A Day at Edgehill: Structured Calm."

So what did I learn from twenty-eight days of "structured calm"? I found out my liver had been damaged, and that if I kept drinking it could turn into cirrhosis. I learned that it was great to laugh without nudging from alcohol. I discovered that sharing feelings—from resentments about my mother to general sadness— was cathartic. Most important, I accepted that, much as it went against every image I had of myself, I was an alcoholic.

Not only did I accept it for myself, I shared it with the public. That is what public people often do, and I had done it before with my drug addiction. But this baring of the soul was especially difficult. I felt like a fraud, having confessed just nineteen months earlier to one addiction while keeping hidden this second one. Yet it was only over the past month that I had admitted it to my- self, and I was spilling my guts this soon after precisely because I could not face the even more imposing burden of another cover- up. I also worried that the public was running out of tolerance for me and that I was again embarrassing my husband, who was serv- ing out the end of his last gubernatorial term and still recovering from his presidential loss.

So I stood before the cameras and uttered those four mortify- ing words: "I am an alcoholic." The reaction was breathtaking, from the press and, more meaningful to me, the from public. I got letters, cards, and calls.* Just eight days after checking out of Edge-

---

*Among the many amazing letters I got when I went public with my addictions was one from Betty Ford, the former First Lady, who suffered her own alcohol and drug dependencies. "My thoughts and prayers are with you," she wrote, "as you discover a new you—one I know you will like and accept as the fine person you are. Sobriety is to know a new joy. Congratulations to you and your husband for openly addressing one of our country's greatest problems."

hill I was off on a national lecture tour talking about my chemical and alcohol dependencies.

Accepting that I was an alcoholic was a vital first step in my recovery, as every recovering alcoholic knows. Talking about it across America helped as well. But neither was enough to keep me from drinking or eliminate the need for more time at treatment clinics. The incident with rubbing alcohol landed me in the intensive care unit at Brigham and Women's Hospital in Boston, then down the street at the psych unit of Deaconess Hospital. The press couldn't get enough of the story once it got the juicy detail about rubbing alcohol, which showed just what a lush I was. One *Globe* reporter I knew and respected played armchair psychiatrist with me and Michael, putting my troubles in the context of his failed bid for the White House: "Despite the ridicule, the governor has not cracked open the door of his feelings even an inch. But Mrs. Dukakis has always been the one family member who was unafraid of showing her emotions, of earning unflattering epithets, such as 'Dragon Lady.' It is not surprising that it is she who could not hide the pain of adjusting to the new, harsh realities of politics and life."

She was right about the pain. When it surfaced again I tried to numb it by swallowing a handful of Tylenol with codeine. The result was another short visit to Deaconess Hospital. My next intensive program was at the Four Winds Psychiatric Hospital in Katonah, New York, where the psychiatrist had enough of a sense of humor to check me in as Abigail Adams. It was the perfect pseudonym. Abigail, like me, had strong opinions on public and private issues of her day, quite apart from those of her opinionated husband John, America's first vice president and second president. She was from my home state of Massachusetts, and as proud of that as I am. And she had a deep, abiding, loving relationship with her husband that helped sustain them both.

That is the sentimental aspect of my arrival at Four Winds in December 1989. The sobering part is how very sick I was then, mentally and physically, as I am reminded by poring over my records from that hospital. "On admission, the patient has physically indicated a precipitous loss of weight, insomnia, inability to concentrate, constant despairing thoughts, feeling a profound sense of hopelessness, a need to be self-punitive, possibly to the point of suicide," wrote Dr. Samuel Klagsbrun, the clinic's medical director. He also described my "constant search for drugs, medications or alcohol to escape her mental state, and over-arching these symptoms a level of guilt and self-loathing that is impossible to lessen and set aside. . . . There is a sense of emptiness and a lack of definition of who she is, compared to the descriptions her family members offer of her. It is as if two people are being described with the patient's description being terribly vague and unstructured."

Worse still, if that is possible, was the doctor's observation that "she"—meaning me—"saw herself as having a disease for which a specific treatment would mechanically cure her of and that she would otherwise be exactly the same person that she had always been. The shallowness of that approach is surprising, if not shocking. Considering the fact that she has had a very public life, the 'as if' style of approaching herself is deeply worrisome." Putting labels to things, the way psychiatrists are wont to do, Klagsbrun said I had major, recurrent depression. I suffered from alcohol abuse, too. I had a "borderline personality disorder with narcissistic, dependent and avoidant feature." And I was in "delayed mourning" over the death of my mother twelve years before.

The solution, the doctor said, was to continue on three drugs: the antidepressant Prozac, the thyroid drug Synthroid, and the estrogen treatment Premarin. He also prescribed daily individual talk therapy, group therapy, and generally taking part in activities on the unit where I would be living. The chance that any of this would make me better, he concluded, was "guarded. The lack of insight and the difficulty in facing up to the reality of her chronic condition makes it questionable to offer a better prognosis at this moment."

Wow. Reading all that, even sixteen years later, takes my breath away. Dr. Klagsbrun was right about how bad I was feeling, whether or not he got the psychiatric jargon right. The good news is that Four Winds combined rigor and gentility, in surroundings as well as treatment approach, in a way that helped me get better. Or at least I was good enough that I could check out and go home two months later.

No one would use a word like "gentle" to describe the Randolph County Hospital in Roanoke, Alabama, where I went after the incident with vanilla extract and hair spray. The Alabama hospital believed in tough love and confronting you with hard truths, which in my case meant drilling in that if I kept up my bad habits I would end up in the morgue. The last place I went for treatment was Massachusetts General Hospital. My stays there were much shorter, generally a few days to dry out. The doctors were caring, sensitive, and discreet, with the latter being especially important since the hospital was practically in my backyard.

Looking back, I can see how much I learned at the addiction clinics and other hospitals. The effect of going to a treatment center is treatment itself, because you are facing up to your need for help. I had a rapport with other people going through the same programs. My doctors, nurses, and fellow patients helped me see how I was slowly eroding away my relationships along with my health. They got me to admit I was a drug addict, a drunk, and a person with severe depression. They put me on antidepressants. Best of all, they got me involved in the international self-help group started by Bill Wilson.

It is called a fellowship, but most people know it by its two-letter acronym. The practice among participants has always been not to talk publicly about the group, or even to name it, because confidentiality is so essential to participation. I don't want to violate that practice here. I can say that I go to meetings once a week. It is ironic that the fellowship is the only treatment program I have not had to pay for, yet it is the one I turn to most often, with greatest effect. My sponsors have become my friends and confidantes. They are there whenever I need them in a way that even the best therapist can't be. Meetings are available in the two cities where I live, Boston and Los Angeles, and anywhere in the world that I am traveling. Once you're in the program, if you take a drink you start again at the beginning. You go back to your home group and start talking about how you had that first drink.

But even the fellowship didn't stop my depression from coming back and dragging me down again. And none of the treatment centers I was at—not Edgehill, where I forged friendships that I still cherish twenty years later, or Hazelden, which I found helpful enough that I went back—could root out my depression. The clinics and programs made me feel better about myself, helping me beat back the amphetamines and, to a lesser but substantial extent, the alcohol. Yet the melancholia was more than they could cope with, or than I could, and had me looking elsewhere for help.

The therapist's couch was one place I looked. I was used to it, having seen psychiatrists at each of my treatment centers and at Boston's Harvard Community Health Plan. In 1998 I started treatment with Dr. Roger Weiss at McLean Hospital, just outside Boston. I continued with him for five years. It was not full-blown Freudian analysis. It was straightforward talk therapy, and at the start it was once a month. Over time it became more irregular. I was traveling a lot, and sometimes we'd do therapy over the

phone. Roger was especially easy for me to talk to since he's a violinist, and he understood instinctively all I was telling him about
my musician-dad. There's nothing I couldn't talk to Roger about.
He knew me so well that we had a context. He was very open
about reminding me of my past behavior, my past reactions. He's
also a fabulous guy, a very gentle man. He specializes in alcohol
issues, alcohol-related depression, which is why I was referred to
him in the first place.

When he heard we were writing this book, Roger agreed to
share his notes from the years I was seeing him, and they reflect
my yo-yo-like ups and down. Literally. There was my fall off a
seawall in Bermuda in the fall of 1998, when I got a concussion
that landed me in the hospital and set off a crying spell. There was
my dozing at the wheel of our car a month later, which scared
Michael even more than me and had me adjust the antidepressants I was taking. Therapy helped me weather those episodes.
Roger also helped me recognize my manic spending sprees, slog
through worrisome drops in libido, and jump back on the wagon
each time I had a drinking binge, which was far too often. Therapy did me a lot of good, but it was not enough. It was great with
sadness, but it was too much to expect that it would silence the
deafening depression.

I also tried a change in scenery and climate. Fall was always a
particularly difficult time for me, probably because I knew a cold
and bleak winter was about to set in. All the attendant pieces of
my depression were present then. Low self-esteem. Feeling I wasn't
attractive, that I wasn't intellectually swift enough to handle all I
had to do. I wanted to be home in my own bedroom. Alone. I had
gone back to school to get my master's in social work, and during
the fall of both those years at Boston University in the mid-1990s
I could barely get myself to study or write the assigned papers. I
tried spending part of every day under a light box in our Brook-

line home, starting as early as July, hoping to head off that autumn's depression. Michael and I tried spending winters in Florida, where he got a teaching job. The sun and warmth helped. Now we spend every winter in Los Angeles. He teaches at UCLA. I work on immigration and other projects, give talks, and spend time with the kids, two of whom live in California. Getting away from the snow and cold of winter, and being nearer my children, gives me a big lift.

Drugs helped a lot, too, at first. Norpramin was my first antidepressant, starting, I think, in 1982, during my first stay at Hazelden. It killed the depression. It also slurred my speech, dried my mouth, made me retain urine, and left me constipated. Along with everyone else, I took Prozac—for about ten years alone, and another six with lithium. It worked, then petered out. I tried Wellbutrin, but it was a nightmare. It made me very anxious, very jiggy. Lithium made me feel doped-up. I just wanted to sleep all the time. I didn't think I was bipolar, but as time went on I began to realize that was my pattern. I'd finish the depression, then have a manic period. For a lot of years I didn't want to admit that was going on because it was so fabulous feeling up after I had been so down. The antidepressant that seemed to work best was Effexor, one of the SSRIs. I stayed on it for about four years. As with the other drugs, my doctors started me on a low dose, then adjusted up to reach the right balance. It sometimes worked in tamping down the depression. It also sometimes made me sleepy, diminished my sexual appetite, and upset my stomach.

Those are the medications I remember. My charts show there were more. I tried a series of antidepressants, from doxepin to desipramine, trazodone, Mirapex, Zoloft, and Remeron. At times I took one drug at a time, but generally it was in combinations. I tried BuSpar, amantadine, and Cylert, each of which the doctors thought might make the Prozac work better. I tried Neurontin, a medication originally used for shingles and seizures that they felt could help with my mania. I tried St.-John's-wort, an herbal remedy for depression. For the last four years, I have used Omega-Brite, a dietary supplement recommended by Dr. Welch that is supposed to promote everything from emotional well-being to cognitive clarity, cardiac and joint health to good digestion.

My records also reflect that each drug was of limited benefit, eventually producing side effects that made me abandon it. "Virtually all prescriptions have been tried but few achieve adequate dose or duration," wrote one of my doctors. Roger Weiss, my therapist, thought the antidepressants might actually have induced the mania. The psychotropic medicines I have taken for nearly twenty-five years generally followed this pattern: They worked for a while, then ran out of power. My son John thinks it is partly Michael's and my fault. We were unrealistic in our expectations, he says, looking for "magic pills—the cocktail of medications that is going to do the trick." The reality, John points out, "is that it's a moving target. If you ever find that magic combination, it's likely not to stay magic for very long."

When my antidepressants couldn't stop the pain and melancholy, there was only one thing that would: alcohol. I had a timeline with my depressions. I would be okay for eight months, then depressed for four. The end of the fourth month was my crisis period. I couldn't cry. I would become anorexic, losing as much as fifteen pounds. I could not concentrate, could not organize things, could not become engaged. I would be so distraught that having a drink was the only way of bringing me away from the terrible feelings I had about myself. I would fall apart and start to drink.

That was the situation facing me when I checked into Massachusetts General Hospital last night, June 19, 2001. I had run out of remedies, and the hospital was the only place I could be sure I wouldn't resort to alcohol. None of those things I worked so hard on—not the pills or the rehabs I had started nineteen years earlier, not the moves or even my self-help program—could keep the cloud from coming back. Each new episode was worse than the one before. The only thing I hadn't tried was the treatment Charlie Welch had discussed with us three long years before. It was a treatment we were disposed to reject, given what it had done to Michael's brother Stelian. It was a last resort, a radical approach we thought had been discarded half a century ago.

So here I am, the morning of my thirty-eighth wedding anniversary, ready to get my first round of electroconvulsive therapy.

Six

IN AND OUT
OF THE CUCKOO'S NEST

If Ugo Cerletti was electroshock's patron saint, Randall Patrick Mc-Murphy was its angel of death.

McMurphy is the bold, brawling roisterer who takes on Nurse Ratched and the rest of the establishment in Ken Kesey's 1962 novel *One Flew Over the Cuckoo's Nest.* Ratched's preferred weapon in taming McMurphy, Kesey tells us, is electric shock, a "device that might be said to do the work of the sleeping pill, the electric chair, *and* the torture rack." The subject is "strapped to a table, shaped, ironically, like a cross," then "five cents' worth of electricity through the brain and you are jointly administered therapy and a punishment for your hostile go-to-hell behavior." For truly recalcitrant patients like McMurphy, treatments are dispensed like aspirin. But he remains stoic even as a nurse sticks a rubber hose between clenched teeth, two robot arms lower soldering irons onto his temples, and the seizure starts. "Light arcs across, stiffens him, bridges him up off the table till nothing is down but his wrists and ankles and out around that crimped black rubber hose a sound like *hooeee!* and he's frosted over completely with sparks."

Enough time in the shock shop, a fellow inmate warns the newly arrived McMurphy, "and a man could turn out like Mr. Ellis you see over there against the wall. A drooling, pants-wetting idiot at thirty-five. . . . Or look at Chief Broom clutching to his namesake there beside you . . . I've heard that the Chief, years ago, received more than two hundred shock treatments when they were really the vogue. Imagine what this could do to a mind that was already slipping. Look at him: a giant janitor."

Kesey's book was hailed by the *New York Times* as a "glittering parable of good and evil" and by *Time* as "a roar of protest against middle-brow society's Rules and the invisible Rulers who enforce them." More adoring still were reviews for Milos Forman's 1975 film adaptation, which quickly became the seventh highest-grossing film ever, won a Best Actor Oscar for Jack Nicholson as McMurphy, and swept all five major Academy Awards for the first time since Frank Capra's 1931 paragon *It Happened One Night*. If they handed out an Oscar for Best Line, it likely would have gone to McMurphy who, upon stumbling out of the ECT room, jokes with his fellow patients, "They was giving me ten thousand watts a day, you know, and I'm hot to trot! The next woman takes me on's gonna light up like a pinball machine and pay off in silver dollars!" His last scene also would have won, for Worst Psychiatric Excess, although all he did was lie on a gurney motionless and emotionless.

Images from the cuckoo's nest were so transfixing that, two generations later, they continue to define public perceptions of shock treatment.

They also are outdated and misleading, and were even when Kesey sketched them in 1962.

In its earliest days, shock treatment did resemble a torture chamber. Patients were pinned to their beds by burly attendants. There was no sedation. Limbs flailed; teeth cracked. But muscle relaxants, anesthesia, and a continuous supply of oxygen all were in regular use by the early 1950s, eliminating the thrashing and belying *Cuckoo's Nest*'s arresting depiction of life in the loony bin. As for McMurphy's final vegetative state, filmgoers could conclude it was the result of a souped-up session of shock when, as Kesey's novel makes clear, it was a by-product of lobotomy.*

Kesey's and Forman's embellishments were partly a reflection of their times. The 1960s and 1970s in America were an era of opening up and sometimes knocking down structures of the state, including mental hospitals. They were too big, too brutal, too much a tool of the establishment. ECT offered an irresistible metaphor for all that was wrong with the asylum. Protestors already were manning the barricades to rage against mind-numbing machines and faraway military interventions. Now they added a new plank, one that called for shuttering shock programs.

One Flew Over the Cuckoo's Nest, the book and movie versions, mirrored those critiques and launched the careers of Kesey and Forman. But the creators of *Cuckoo's Nest* did more than reflect the age's excesses. They stoked them by depicting electroshock as what Kesey calls "a clever little procedure, simple, quick, nearly painless it happens so fast, but no one ever wants another one. Ever." No hint of its benefits. No sense that doctors and nurses were after anything but punishment, or that some patients actually wanted the treatment. No bounds on artistic license. Forman's and Kesey's stigmatizing sketches, like those of fellow writers and filmmakers, were seared into the public mind. They help explain why, by 1980, use of shock treatment had plummeted by 50 percent from just five years before, with many state psychiatric hospitals abandoning it outright.

It was one of the most precipitous collapses ever for a trusted medical remedy—and perhaps the only one that happened as evidence was building that it worked and its risks could be reduced. Medical journals published shock's obituary, fewer and fewer psychiatrists were being

---

*Forman's film did include two close-ups of the scars on McMurphy's head, but it took a viewer who was medically savvy or had read Kesey's book to realize those were the marks of lobotomy surgery.

trained to administer it, and, by 1983, thirty-two states had approved legal restrictions. After being admonished in 1950 that it would be a crime if they did not offer electroshock to their sickest patients, psychiatrists thirty years later worried that it could be a crime if they did.

∽○

Not all of electroshock's traumas came at the hands of writers and moviemakers. Shock doctors undermined their own credibility and their therapy's by prescribing it for conditions where it does not work. As recently as the early 1970s, people with neuroses made up as much as a quarter of the electroshock caseload in some hospitals, despite a stack of scientific reports making clear that it was not helpful and could actually harm them. It was also given as a first-line treatment for persistent schizophrenia long after that prescription was cast in doubt. Other applications never had any rational roots, but that did not stop doctors from trying to shock back into normalcy patients who had head injuries, back pain, asthma, or psoriasis. Then there was the case, reported by the *New York Times* in 1948, of "an unmarried 20-year-old girl who stammered so badly that she could speak only in occasional monosyllables." After thirteen shock sessions at a West Virginia clinic, the girl "now talks freely and even sings."

Doubts about such "promiscuous and indiscriminate" applications were raised as early as 1947 by a distinguished collection of physicians who called themselves the Group for the Advancement of Psychiatry. "The evidence is conflicting as to its efficacy in the schizophrenias," GAP advised, while "the preponderance of evidence indicates that the use of electro-shock therapy is contra-indicated in the psychoneuroses." These psychiatrists understood that while researchers were beginning to document the kinds of cases where ECT did and did not work, word was slow to filter back to practitioners. And they worried that electroshock could easily suffer the same fate as earlier remedies du jour like

Metrazol and malaria therapy, falling faster than it rose. The way to fore-stall that was not to brush aside the "widespread abuses" in its usage, but to face them head-on. So concerned was GAP that it threatened to sound an alarm and, in a move unimaginable in polite medical society, to push for limits on the procedure.

Looking back today, Dr. Matthew Rudorfer, the National Institute of Mental Health's top official overseeing ECT and related treatments, says GAP was right. It saw, at the crest of ECT's gilded era, seeds of dark days to come. The blame, he explains, lies less with electroshock practitioners than with the wider profession: "The field of psychiatry really lagged be-hind the rest of medicine in terms of standards. It was less evidence-based, there was a long reliance on theory rather than data." That was the case in the late 1800s and early 1900s, when psychoanalysis was the gold standard and was used to treat conditions where it was worthless as well as ones where it could help. It remained the case in the mid–1900s, when ECT filled that niche and "was used for everything under the sun," adds Rudorfer. "There were no other good options. In some ways, ECT never recovered because it was used sometimes quite inappropriately."

Other times the diagnosis was appropriate, but too many treatments were given at too punishing a dose. One patient was given 800 sessions. Another got 248 over three years. A half dozen with schizophrenia re-ceived between 110 and 234 shocks each. Reports of piling on like that piled up in medical journals and the popular press beginning in the 1940s and continuing through the 1970s. At first the thinking was intuitive: use as much as it takes to get someone well. Eventually, a whole school of re-search and rationalization developed that certain intensely ill patients needed more intensive therapy. Dr. Lucio Bini, Cerletti's collaborator in founding electroshock, in 1942 described his approach of administering several sessions a day of shock, dubbing it Annihilation. Others called it by the equally alarming appellations of Confusional Treatment and Blitz Electric Shock Therapy (when writing about the latter, its adherents wisely opted for its acronym, BEST). The most descriptive title, and the one that stuck, was Regressive Electroshock Treatment (again, its boosters preferred a more soothing mnemonic, REST).

REST meant inducing two to four grand mal seizures a day, five to seven days a week, until "regression" was achieved. "Regression is assumed to be complete," one set of authors wrote in 1957, "when the patient manifests a majority of the following signs: There are memory loss, marked confusion, disorientation, lack of verbal spontaneity, slurring of speech to the point of complete dysarthria or muteness, and utter apathy. The patient behaves like a helpless infant, is incontinent in both bowel and bladder functions, requires spoon-feeding and, at times, tube-feeding. Frequently, he holds his food in his mouth as if unaware that he should swallow it—permitting fluids to flow out of the mouth." Sending a patient into that regressed state, then letting him slowly emerge, alters his brain in a way that releases him from the shackles of schizophrenia and other disabling diseases. Or at least that is the way early boosters said it worked with their patients, who included "teachers, chemists, graduate students, priests, and a rabbi." Their results looked impressive, much the way early findings had for sleep therapy, insulin coma, and even lobotomies. Overusing a therapy in its embryonic days is hardly unusual; it happened with hysterectomies and tonsillectomies. But over time psychiatrists realized that regression is not only antithetical to a good ECT response, it produces serious memory loss. They also recoiled at the idea of putting patients through the anguish and danger of a treatment that is anything but REST—and at the premise that more is better with shock treatment. "Regressive ECT," the National Institutes of Health announced definitively if belatedly in 1985, "is no longer an acceptable treatment form."

It also is no longer appropriate to use electroshock to punish or control patients, and never was. Yet that happened often enough to encourage Kesey's one-dimensional portrait of the cuckoo's nest as a hotbed of heavy-handed social control. A 1960 report of interviews with nurses and attendants who administered electroshock offered a window into those practices. "When patients are combative, destructive, and violent they need to go on treatment and get some of that knocked out of them," one staffer testified. At the midcentury mark the Milledgeville asylum in Georgia, the world's biggest mental hospital, was administering three thousand shock treatments a year. Superintendent T. G. Peacock acknowledged that it was "hospital policy to use *shock treatment* to insure good citizenship." It also was policy, with just fifteen doctors for ten thousand patients, to run the shock room like an assembly line where "patients were not prepared either psychologically or with drugs for treatment, and except for a supervised coma after treatment, they were left to walk stuporously back to the day room, confused but quiet and amenable to being herded by the meekest attendant." Milledgeville staff had a special name for the electroshock they dispensed so freely as therapy and punishment: a "Georgia Power Cocktail."

At most asylums the lines between therapy, control, and punishment were more blurred than at Milledgeville, reflecting psychiatrists' intent to serve their patients but also their resolution to keep command of the institution. Those nuances come alive in Dr. Joel Braslow's exhaustive review of records from the 1940s and 1950s at the huge Stockton State Hospital in California. "First, physicians believed in electroshock as an integral part of their scientific discipline, a modern therapeutic practice," Braslow writes. "Second, physicians used electroshock therapy as a medical form of corporal discipline, a means to control undesirable/ diseased behaviors via the body. Third, when used properly, they saw this practice as unassailably therapeutic: the control of bodies was the control of disease."

That push-pull of the shock doctor as caring therapist *and* controlling overseer was there from the inauguration of the therapy. Was Maestro Cerletti an arrogant researcher or a pioneering healer when he ignored his patient S.E.'s plea that another dose could kill him? Surely a bit of both. "Such explicit admonition under such circumstances, and so emphatic and commanding, coming from a person whose enigmatic jargon had until then been very difficult to understand, shook my determination to carry on with the experiment," Cerletti himself later acknowledged. "But it was just this fear of yielding to a superstitious notion that caused me to make up my mind. The electrodes were applied again."* The same question of motives can be asked of another electroshock pioneer, Dr. Abram Bennett, who admitted in 1949 that "we prefer to explain as little as possible to the uninformed patient." He was rightfully trying to calm his patients' anxieties, realizing, as he said, that "even use of the terms 'shock,' 'convulsion,' etc., are often traumatic." He also was exhibiting the hubris of doctor knows best that was standard practice then, in the process violating his patients' basic right to know.

Ellen Field experienced firsthand the tension between shock as therapy and as restraint. "Except for the minority who yelled, kicked, and screamed, most of us suffered inwardly in the realization that we had no defense, and that resistance would be sure to get us a stronger treatment," she wrote in a 1964 memoir. "A news photographer could take a picture of shock treatment morning on our ward, and everything would look calm. But from the subjective angle (i.e., horizontal angle), it looks like an Alfred Hitchcock movie where some horror is present invisibly while ordinary visible things move along normally. . . . These givers of this brutal assault are impervious to human feelings."

Field was not unusual in those early decades of electroshock in having little say over when, how, or whether she was treated. Involuntary admission was much more commonplace then, and patients were forced to take whatever therapy doctors opted for. At Stockton State, Braslow found that a mere 22 percent of shock patients had agreed to the treatment. Robert Whitaker, author of the exposé *Mad in America,* estimates

---

*In a moment of even greater candor, Cerletti admitted that "when subjecting unconscious patients to such an extremely violent reaction as these convulsions, I had a sense of illicitness and felt as though I had somehow betrayed these patients."

that more than 1 million patients received "forced electroshock" in the 1940s and 1950s.

Issues of consent are especially vexing when the patient is a child as young as four and the shock is administered as many as forty times. That happened in an experiment at Bellevue Hospital in the mid-1940s. Ninety-eight children diagnosed with severe schizophrenia, one just four years old and all under twelve, were shocked once a day every day but Sunday. The total typically was twenty treatments, although in some cases it ran to forty. The trial lasted five years. It was the first serious attempt to use ECT on prepubescent youth, and it sparked a debate that is still raging sixty years later about safety, image, and effectiveness. Electroshock left the children "less disturbed, less excitable, less withdrawn, and less anxious," Lauretta Bender, the study's director, wrote in 1947. Her tests, she said, also proved that "children can tolerate electric shock better than adults." But Bender acknowledged that ECT did nothing to help her young subjects adapt emotionally, think clearly, express themselves, or ease the other symptoms of childhood schizophrenia for which they were being treated.

Researchers at another New York hospital offered an even bleaker picture of Bender's experiment based on follow-up treatment and testing of thirty of the Bellevue children. Fewer than a third of the children actually were schizophrenic, while a few others were psychopathic, doctors at Rockland State Hospital wrote in 1954. The rest merely had behavior disorders. As for whether shock worked over the longer run, they pointed to several instructive cases. A nine-year-old boy tried to hang himself because he thought he might get more shock treatment, was "afraid of dying," and "wanted to get it over with fast." An eight-year-old boy attempted to strangle his sister. A seven-year-old girl beat her infant brother. Overall, the Rockland doctors concluded, "the effects of [ECT] were temporary, and resulted in no sustained improvement in the patterning of behavior. Relapses occurred in all cases, necessitating continued hospitalization."

For the field of ECT, the Bellevue study set back attempts to use electroshock on young people of any age. In retrospect, it is clear that Bender was too quick to lump any child with tantrums, fantasies, and other troublesome symptoms as schizophrenic, although the whole psychiatric profession was doing that in those days, with adults and children. It also is clear that twenty shock treatments in less than a month is too much.* What is less clear is just when ECT is appropriate for people with schizophrenia, or for children.

For Ted Chabasinski, the Bellevue study was life-shattering. Chabasinski was one of Bender's ninety-eight children, and one of the Rockland thirty. At age six he was removed from his foster home and committed to the pediatric psychiatric ward at Bellevue. His "condition," he says, was a family history of mental disease that had his social worker and others seeing illness in him when he was just behaving like a kid. The "solution" was electroshock. Chabasinski cannot remember details of his sessions, but he does recall "them jamming this handkerchief in my mouth and it making me choke." Looking back is still painful for the sixty-eight-year-old lawyer, who calls Bender's work "a complete denial of humanity" and compares it to experiments carried out by the Nazis and to lynchings of blacks in the American South. His experience as a child made him into a lifelong opponent of electroshock. On the one hand, he believes people should be free to choose that or any other treatment they want. On the other, he says, "there are all kinds of terrible drugs out there that we don't allow them to have. Why should shock be any different?"

---

*Bender went on to give shock treatments to even younger patients, one of whom, named Bert, was two years and ten months old when he had the first of his twenty sessions. She also gave the hallucinogen LSD to schizophrenic children, as young as six, on a daily basis for six weeks. Her subjects, she reported, were happier, less aggressive, healthier physically, and more responsive to other children and to adults.

Chabasinski and other critics did not just ruminate over their concerns. They pressed them with politicians, journalists, and the public, helping launch an anti-ECT movement in California that spread east, then south, then overseas.

It was the perfect moment. The 1960s and 1970s were the eras of agitation in America. There was the movement against the Vietnam War and the movement for women's liberation. The New Left was born. Civil rights was capturing its most coveted prizes. The Great Society declared a War on Poverty, and President Richard Nixon declared one on cancer. New York's Stonewall Riots gave birth to a Gay Power insurrection. John, Paul, George, and Ringo, with a little help from their friends Timothy Leary and Bob Dylan, were shaping a counterculture that was all for experimenting with drugs, sex, and Eastern religions, and was heart and soul against what outgoing president Dwight D. Eisenhower had branded the military-industrial complex.

A number of narrower movements sprouted at the same time that became lightning rods for the era's idealism and ferment. The crusade against nuclear power was one. The battle against electric shock therapy was another. Shock resonated because, like nuclear energy, it had the aura of an out-of-control technology imposed by an authoritarian society. Such critiques might have had limited appeal in the feel-good 1950s or the high-tech 1990s, when faith ran high in the capacity of machines to relieve stress as well as promote prosperity. But they touched a nerve in the social upheaval that commenced in the 1960s. Mental asylums were convincingly painted as places that restrained creativity and exercised control. Psychiatry was running amok, the critics charged, and what better proof than its use of a tortuous treatment like electric shock?

Around the same time, media reports were pouring in from Hungary, Russia, Australia, and Argentina of electroshock's use in real torture. In

Canada, psychiatrist D. Ewen Cameron got CIA funds in the 1950s to run a series of brainwashing experiments. Without telling his patients they were guinea pigs, he used high-dose ECT, hallucinogenic drugs, sensory deprivation, and barbiturate-induced sleep to try to obliterate neurotic ideas, replacing them with messages of his choosing. He thought the approach would be therapeutic. CIA officials thought it would let them understand the brainwashing techniques used by America's cold war enemies and perhaps counter with their own form of mind control. Cameron's patients could hardly think. The experiments left them dazed, incontinent, and oftentimes in utter terror. In Indonesia, meanwhile, everyone's intent was to treat mental disorders, but the primitive technology that hospitals used in 1959 looked like torture. Two electrodes were strapped to the patient's head, then, at a nod from the doctor, a nurse plugged the other end of the cord directly into the wall outlet. There was no shock machine to control the safety of the current or its duration. At a second sign from the doctor, the nurse unplugged the cord, the patient had a seizure, and all was presumed to be well.

One way activists sought to strike back at those forces of technology and terror was to deinstitutionalize and decentralize social structures—from prisons to the Pentagon, schools, and, most of all, huge madhouses. A series of disparate groups came together to say "no"—to organized psychiatry and to electroshock. Some were psychiatrists disillusioned by their profession's inclination to impose solutions on patients and its insistence on using a "brain-disabling" treatment like shock. The father of the antipsychiatry movement was Dr. Thomas Szasz, a Budapest-born, Chicago-trained psychoanalyst who laid out his gospel in his 1960 book *The Myth of Mental Illness.* It was simple and enticing: Mental disease is an invention of a controlling society, manipulative relatives, and conniving psychiatrists. Picking up on that theme was Dr. Peter Roger Breggin, author of *Electroshock: Its Brain-Disabling Effects* and a hero of the anti-ECT movement. Students and other reformers joined in, seeing ECT as the incarnation of Kesey's all-controlling Combine and Eisenhower's military-industrial behemoth. Scientologists got involved in 1969 by founding the formidable Citizens Commission on Human Rights, which argues that electroshock is "as scientific as sticking one's head in a light socket."*

The moral center of the new movement was Chabasinski and his fellow "survivors." They saw themselves as having outlasted a mental health system with brutally flawed solutions, most notably shock treatment, and as launching a struggle for civil rights as vital as those being waged by blacks, gays, and women. The consumer mental health movement they helped spawn is today more mainstream and broad-based, with a less monolithic and antagonistic position on ECT and a wider human rights agenda. But back then electric shock was the primary symbol and target. In Portland, Oregon, the critics crowned themselves the Insane Liberation Front. In New York it was the Mental Patients Liberation Project. And in California, the center of the storm over ECT as it has been with other social movements, they united under the Network Against Psychiatric Assault. Leonard Roy Frank, a linchpin of the California juggernaut, explains that "our lives had been diminished because of electroshock." In his case that meant getting fifty insulin coma treatments and thirty-five shocks during an involuntary commitment in 1962 and 1963, in the process losing more than two years of memories to the point where "I

---

*Scientology and its offshoots are among the most unremitting enemies of ECT and its practitioners, calling it "pain inflicted in the name of therapy" and branding them liars and abusers. But L. Ron Hubbard, Scientology's founder, took a considerably softer tone in *Dianetics*, his 1950 book that spells out the tenets of his faith. Referring to psychiatrists who perform electroshock and even lobotomy, Hubbard wrote, "A witch-burning attitude toward these people is very far from the one adopted by Dianetics. Pointing to the fact that they have murdered minds which would otherwise have recovered, labeling them 'mind snatchers,' and making a horror story out of their actions is far from rational conduct. On the whole, these people have been entirely sincere in their efforts to help the insane."

didn't even know the president of the United States was John Kennedy. I use the expression ECB, electroconvulsive brainwashing. It cleans out those ideas that are inappropriate for a person to have in our culture."

He was not the only one who felt robbed. Others were beginning to tell their stories—of ECT administered for conditions where it offered little help, of too many treatments delivered at too high doses, and especially of being shocked against their will. Those were precisely the issues that the Group for the Advancement of Psychiatry and other reformers from within the mental health community had warned about a generation before. But no one was listening that far back. Few former patients were out of the closet then; fewer still were sounding off. American medicine and American society were less self-critical than they would be later. ECT was still king in the 1940s, 1950s, and into the 1960s, and hardly anyone was ready to talk truth to power.

By the 1970s, Frank and his California compatriots were ready enough to explode. They picketed outside electroshock clinics with signs linking the practitioners to Spanish inquisitor Tomás de Torquemada and Nazi executioner Adolf Eichmann. They staged a sleep-in at the office of Governor Jerry Brown. They published then, and still do, a "Shock Doctor Roster" that parodies those doctors' daily rosters of patients. Opponents also did a masterful job linking electric shock therapy with that most Draconian of mental remedies, lobotomy. Surgically removing or destroying part of their brain does calm distraught patients—often at the price of their personalities and even their lives. Lobotomies had little connection to ECT, relying on surgery rather than electricity, disabling rather than convulsing the brain, and fading into disuse in the mid-1950s as electroshock was entering its heyday. But its barbarous image was too potent to resist for antipsychiatry guru Dr. Peter Breggin. ECT and lobotomy "both cause brain tissue damage," Breggin wrote in 1979. "Both are aimed at the control of thoughts, feelings, and actions; and both are applied to persons who have no disease of the brain."

Tactics like those touched a nerve and engendered action. In 1974,

California passed the nation's most restrictive law on ECT. When it was struck down as unconstitutional in 1976, another law was passed banning the treatment for anyone under age twelve, requiring two doctors to concur even with voluntary patients, and ordering the state to record everything from shocks administered to cases where memory loss was reported. Doctors intentionally breaking the law, which is still in effect, can be fined $10,000 per violation and lose their license.

ECT critics were encouraged but not satisfied. Electroshock had to be stopped. If the state would not do it, localities might. What better city to try first than Berkeley, birthplace of the Free Speech Movement and home to one of the region's biggest shock programs. A Coalition to Stop Electroshock was formed, chaired by Chabasinski and bringing together everyone from the mayor to leftist activists and blacks upset that so many in their community were getting forced treatment at state mental hospitals. An antishock initiative was put on the ballot in 1982 and widely covered by the national and local press. In November, Berkeley residents voted nearly two to one to make ECT a crime punishable by six months in jail or a $500 fine. While a court quickly overturned the ordinance, its supporters had delivered a resounding message: Electroshock is a political time bomb; users beware.

ECT doctors heard the warning, and some stopped offering the treatment. So did some hospitals, especially public ones. Newly mandated state records confirmed that California's rate of using ECT was less than half that nationally, with one researcher who examined the decline concluding that "complex legal regulation bears much of the responsibility." A pair of UCLA doctors wrote about their patients who, because state law requires a court order for involuntary ECT, were not able to get treated in time. One was a desperately manic twenty-one-year-old man who had to wait twenty-two days for court approval. He got his ECT and recovered, but his "final two weeks in the hospital were spent reliving the horror of the waiting period," the UCLA team reported, adding that the patient told them he "felt like an animal, tied up, urinating on myself."

The doctors were unable to get a court okay to give ECT to another involuntary patient, a twenty-three-year-old woman with recurrent mania, and within a month she died of cardiac arrest. That "untimely death," the UCLA physicians concluded, "is an apt, albeit extreme example of how the new law may have the overall effect of harming rather than helping the patient."

The California experience spawned imitators across the country, with journalists writing about ECT excesses and critics pressing for change. The *New York Times,* in a 1977 editorial entitled "States' Rights vs. Victims' Rights," asked readers to "imagine (and these are real-life cases, typifying conditions in several states) having a relative in a public mental hospital and learning he had been subjected to electric shock treatment 800 times. . . . There are one million Americans in public institutions— jails and prisons and homes and hospitals for children, the retarded, the elderly. They are, in a way, the most vulnerable Americans. Why can they not be systematically protected against electrodes or cockroaches or rape?" State legislators read editorials like that, linking ECT to roaches and rape, and responded with one restrictive law after another. Some set controls on involuntary treatment. Others went further, limiting the right to consent to ECT. Nearly every state now has some sort of restraint. Colorado bans the treatment for anyone under sixteen. So does Texas, which has even stricter reporting requirements than California. The Lone Star State requires that patients be informed of the treatment's "significant risks" and the "division of opinion as to the efficacy of the procedure," and limits to twenty-four the number of treatments given during any twelve-month period.* Idaho lets doctors doing an emergency evaluation of a child administer drugs or any other treatment they

---

*While the number of patients getting ECT in Texas has gradually climbed back since the law took effect, a senior state official says the number of hospitals offering the treatment has "definitely declined dramatically, and the number of doctors providing it has gone down as well."

think is needed, except ECT, and under nonemergency circumstances it invests the power to approve ECT for a child not in the parents but in a judge. No ECT has been done in a state hospital there, on a child or adult, for at least thirty years. Missouri lets a court order ECT for an unwilling patient only after showing that "there is no less drastic alternative form of therapy which could lead to substantial improvement in the patient's condition," and it bans it for the mentally retarded. Utah, which passed the nation's first ECT statute in 1967, prohibits it for anyone who is under eighteen or pregnant.

Critics also pushed the Food and Drug Administration to probe the safety of ECT devices. They pointed out that the machines had been exempted from rigorous new federal review when the FDA started regulating medical equipment in 1976, partly because ECT devices had been around for so long and because the agency presumed they were safe and effective. FDA responded by waffling, at times suggesting it was about to declare ECT machines safe, at least for severe depression, then hinting at tougher regulation. In the end the agency let manufacturers continue selling their product provided it put out no more energy than ECT machines prior to passage of the 1976 law. That upset critics who insisted the old machines were unsafe, and practitioners who say the dose of those devices is barely half what some patients require and what is available in models sold overseas. In one of the agency's rare moments of candor on the issue, FDA commissioner Donald Kennedy wrote in a 1979 letter to a college professor, "The classification of ECT has become the most controversial proposal of the neurological device series."

Even better evidence of how controversial ECT had become, and how stigmatized, came in the summer of 1972, when Democratic presidential nominee George McGovern picked as his running mate Senator Thomas F. Eagleton of Missouri. Less than two weeks after their nominating convention, Eagleton disclosed that he had a history of "nervous exhaustion" and had twice gotten electric shock. "There is in the minds of some people a stigma attached to any kind of an emotional situation,"

Eagleton told a hall packed with reporters at McGovern's vacation retreat. With his wife Barbara next to him and a slight tic visible in his
hands and face, Eagleton declared himself "very relieved that after living
with this for twelve years, it's now a matter of public record and the people
can judge, as they see fit, as to whether I'm a competent public official."

The American people never got to render their judgment. McGovern at first backed the Missouri senator "1,000 percent," but six days
later he dropped Eagleton from the ticket. Admitting depression was one
thing, but the fallout from confessing to shock treatment was too onerous to overcome in the opinion of the McGovern camp and most political analysts. Missouri voters, who knew Eagleton better, returned him
to the Senate for two more terms.*

The same forces aligned against ECT in the United States were at
work across Europe, oftentimes carrying a more ferocious wallop. In Germany, researchers in 1987 tried to sort out why electroshock was given to
just one of every fifty patients who potentially could benefit from it, a
rate even lower than California's and less than a quarter of that in Denmark and Great Britain. The primary reason, they concluded, is "the recent attacks in the media that presented ECT as a symbol of an inhuman
and repressive form of psychiatry, a deliberate piece of misinformation to
the public. These attacks certainly have had an impact on patients who
expected to receive a frightening and alleged brain-damaging treatment
when ECT was recommended, as well as on some psychiatrists who
adopted the same misconceptions."

In Italy, where Cerletti pioneered the procedure, the attacks found an
even more receptive audience. In 1978, not long after California had

---

*Asked in 2005 what he thought about the whole episode, the seventy-five-year-old Ea-
gleton replied by e-mail, saying, "I had shock treatment in the first half of the 1960s. I
have not kept up with medical science trends in shock treatment, but I know a couple of
highly regarded psychiatrist friends who speculate that it has fallen into disfavor and that I
would not have had such a treatment in the 21st century. By the way, I have not had a depression since the mid-1960s."

rewritten its ECT laws, feminists in Italy joined with students and leftists to successfully press for the dismantlement of most psychiatric hospitals. Care for the mentally ill, they insisted, should be community-based and "demedicalized." Within this broader assault on traditional mental health care, ECT stood as a powerful symbol of psychiatric abuse, much as it did in America. Whatever psychiatrists thought about the procedure, it was taboo for them to prescribe or even discuss it. It remains nearly impossible to get the treatment today in Italy, where it is banned as a means of achieving "rapid remission of [psychiatric] symptoms" and allowed only under a very narrowly prescribed set of circumstances.

∽

At the same time it was under assault by critics outside psychiatry, ECT was being dealt a near-fatal drubbing from within.

Electroshock held a virtual monopoly through the mid-1950s. It was the sole therapy trusted to treat the most severe of the mentally ill, be they in the back wards of mental asylums or attic bedrooms. Psychotherapy could help with neuroses and other emotional disorders, but generally not with ones that were more chemically based and more disabling. Metrazol and insulin were increasingly giving way to electrically induced shocks. Lobotomies had never gained a firm foothold.

Miracle medicines were the trust-busters. Doctors had been using drugs to treat mental ailments since the Middle Ages, with little precision or impact. Laxatives were given on the theory that poisons backed up in the colon could make people crazy. Sedatives calmed the agitated; narcotics lifted the depressed. But the drug that kicked off the psychopharmaceutical revolution was chlorpromazine, or Thorazine, the name pharmaceutical giant Smith Kline & French used in bringing the medication to the United States in the spring of 1954. Thorazine did for psychoses what Viagra would do for impotence, educating America about an ailment as well as a hopeful new approach to treatment. It also opened the floodgates to other wonder drugs: Tofranil and Elavil for depression, lithium for mania, Prolixin and Haldol for psychoses. All were founded on the notion that the mind operates according to the same biological and chemical principles as the rest of the body. With science as their rationale and money as their motivation, drug companies kept the medications coming through the 1960s and 1970s. Psychotropics were prescribed to tens of thousands of patients, then hundreds of thousands, and eventually millions. Many if not most would have been candidates for electroshock just a few years earlier, just as many of the drug-dispensing doctors would have been dispensing ECT. Much as electroshock had supplanted Metrazol, which had displaced insulin coma, which outlasted sleep therapy, so ECT now was being pushed aside by the compelling and consummately American prospect of swallowing a pill to resolve psychological woes.

Psychotherapy also experienced a revival in the 1960s and 1970s, although not on the scale of the drug boom. Freud was an icon on college campuses, where his writings formed the core of syllabuses not just in psychology courses but sociology and even political science. Child-rearing advice from the Austrian analyst's devotee Dr. Benjamin Spock had become the bible for young parents. And millions of Americans a year were visiting psychoanalysts, psychologists, and social workers. Psychotherapy posed less direct competition to ECT than psychopharmaceuticals, because the two generally treat different conditions. Yet therapists were too busy with their practices, and too worried about their own rivalry with the new world of pill popping, to stand up for ECT.

Did the wonder drugs live up to their billing? They did if you were running a mental hospital and trying to get through the day. "The wild, screaming, unapproachable patient was a thing of the past" by the late 1950s thanks to medications like Thorazine, reserpine, and Dilantin, recalled Bliss Forbush, a former president of Baltimore's esteemed Sheppard and Enoch Pratt Hospital. "Attempts at escape were reduced, and serious attempts at suicide less frequent. With the aid of tranquilizers, many more patients could go for drives in the country, visit Towson and Baltimore for shopping excursions, with or without attendants, go to the theatre, visit art museums, take in athletic contests." From patients' perspective, too, things often seemed better. Some saw their demons disappear. Many more, hundreds of thousands, were released from the asylum to the community not just for excursions but for good, their symptoms calmed or at least disguised by drugs, their release saving the public money and making it less anxious about the detested nuthouse.

But as early as the 1950s, researchers had worried that Thorazine generated the same shuffling gait and masklike face as Parkinson's disease, along with sluggishness, jaundice, dry mouth, and hypertension. Its sister drugs had their own hidden curses, blunting emotions, slowing movement, spurring anxiety, and sometimes ending in violent outbursts. Worst of all, the new psychotropics failed to work at all for one in five patients who took them, and over the course of years stopped working for even more.

None of those reservations took hold in the early years of the drug revolution. Patients and doctors were too bewitched by the pills' promise, just as they had been with insulin coma, Metrazol, and electroshock. Anyone disillusioned with one drug, say Geigy's antidepressant Tofranil, did not have long to wait for a rival drugmaker like Merck to unveil a potentially better product like Elavil. Some really were better; others were "me too" drugs synthesized to mimic the big sellers. Much the way ECT was overused in its early years, with problems minimized if not denied, so were the new psychiatric medicines seen as a panacea. Sales soared, and by 1970, Thorazine alone was raking in $116 million a year in profits. Drugmakers used those windfalls to ply with favors the doctors, medical societies, press, and politicians who were key to their continued success. All of which kept doctors writing prescriptions and patients filling them.

ECT had no such benefactors. The only companies making a profit off the therapy were manufacturers of shock machines, of which there are now just two in America. Those devices cost about $12,000 each, and in a great year each company might sell 150, yielding a profit that device makers say is barely $100,000. Compare that to the $35 billion that the ten biggest drug companies earn a year. What that means now and meant back then is that while drugmakers have all the money they need to develop new products, nearly all ECT research has depended on meager allotments from the government. And while drug companies spend tens of billions of dollars a year to market and advertise their wares, ECT companies spend next to nothing. "ECT is not profitable to industry," writes psychiatrist and *Washington Post* columnist Keith Russell Ablow. "If it were, there might be a flurry of industry-supported research to document its effectiveness and reduce its stigma. Psychiatrists would get the same hard-sell education materials on ECT as we do on antidepressants. Maybe even some pens, pads of paper and briefcases with little lightning bolts or something, just like the ones we get with drug logos. But it's the power company that is paid for electric current, not a pharmaceutical manufacturer."

Electroshock might have been able to overcome its excesses, its critics, even its pharmaceutical rivals, if it had been left alone to battle it out on the merits. But it was far too tempting a target for filmmakers, authors, and journalists to leave alone.

They were drawn first by what one psychiatrist calls ECT's Unholy Trinity: electricity, convulsion, and memory loss. Each conjures up frightful images; multiply by three and you have a ready-made horror film, exposé, or the beginning of an alluring novel. Psychiatrists should have been especially sensitive to how troubling such symbols would be in a world where toddlers are conditioned to never, ever put their fingers near a socket, where epileptics are treated like lepers, and where the scariest disease of all is memory-robbing Alzheimer's. But instead of downplaying them, doctors unconsciously highlighted electroshock's vulnerabilities. How else to explain describing the therapy's intensive regimens as Annihilation, Confusion, Blitz, and Regression—names dreamed up not by those treatments' critics but by their authors? Or for Cerletti to opt in the first instance for a term as power-packed and poisonous as electroshock. He and his fellow founders had tin ears to public perception that are unimaginable in today's spin-saturated society. The pioneers eventually did recognize their folly and over the years contemplated renaming the procedure electrofit, electroplexy, clonotherapy, electrically induced convulsions, and even electroshake. Sometime in the 1970s they settled on the slightly more reassuring label of electroconvulsive therapy. Better still, its antiseptic acronym: ECT.

By then it was too late. Whatever the doctors called it, headline writers for the next thirty years would revert back to loaded words like "shock" to make their point and grab their readers. Novelists and filmmakers had already been drawn in and laid out their own story lines.

ECT's silver-screen debut came in the 1948 movie *The Snake Pit,* an adaptation of Mary Jane Ward's 1946 novel of the same name. It was a breakthrough in its sobering, illuminating look at life inside an asylum, earning six Oscar nominations. But it was a portentous beginning for ECT. The treatment is portrayed as punishment, one in a series that heroine Virginia Cunningham endures, including hydrotherapy, drug-induced psychoanalysis, and banishment to the "snake pit," an enormous room where the most psychotic patients engage and enrage one another. When Virginia's husband hears she is about to be shocked, he asks the doctor, "Do you have to? Isn't there any other way?" Virginia pleads, "You're going to electrocute me? Was my crime so great. . . . They're going to kill me without a trial." The sense of doom builds as the camera zooms in on the luminous dials of the ECT machine. Three nurses hold Virginia down, and trumpets join with flutes in building to the crescendo of the seizure itself.

The film's real drama, which is given little buildup or ballyhoo, is that a series of shock treatments leave Virginia well enough to productively participate in psychotherapy, and later to go home with her husband.

The next movie, *Fear Strikes Out*, was the fairest shake electroshock would get from Hollywood. That may be because it was released in 1957, during the therapy's Golden Age, or because ECT really helped Jimmy Piersall, the Boston Red Sox slugger portrayed by Anthony Perkins. Facing unremitting pressure to perform from his father, Piersall suffers a catatonic breakdown and ends up on a mental ward. "We've tried almost everything," the doctor explains to Piersall's wife. "There's only one other possibility. I need your consent for that, electroshock." The music this time is soothing, and the procedure is pictured more like therapy than torture. The clear implication is that it works, at least for Piersall.

With the dawn of the 1960s and electroshock's slow fall from grace, movies became less kind and less nuanced. In *Shock Corridor* (1963), a reporter who goes into a mental hospital undercover is held down by attendants as a rolled-up towel is stuffed into his mouth. He screams for his girlfriend as electricity courses through his wide-awake body. Scary image, the more so if it were true. In fact, the reporter would have blacked out before having a seizure whether or not he got anesthesia and muscle relaxant, and, by 1963, he would have gotten both. In *A Woman Under the Influence* (1974) and *Frances* (1982), shock is used to buck up prevailing social norms and squelch renegades and rebels. There were even comedies like *The Beverly Hillbillies* (1993), where Granny is shocked until her hair stands straight up and sparks fly from her head.

The big screen could not seem to get enough of ECT, with twenty-two films featuring the treatment between 1948 and the turn of the century, and more coming out every year. Part of the appeal was psychiatric sickness itself, which makes for heartrending plots. But Hollywood needs histrionics. And while many more mentally ill people are treated with drugs than electroshock, it is difficult to imagine even Alfred Hitchcock squeezing drama out of a patient popping a pill.

Two Australian psychiatrists analyzed every film they could find with ECT in it, and every aspect of the treatment's depiction. Their conclusion: "ECT is not portrayed with authenticity." Whereas most psychiatrists are avuncular, in the movies they become "cruel, the embodiment of evil." ECT is generally used to treat depression or psychosis; in Hollywood it is "prescribed to overcome antisocial behavior." Anesthesia has been a standard since the 1950s, but "films show patients fully awake and in terror." Study after study, the Australians write, shows that ECT helps most patients, but if they get it on the big screen they end up in a "confused zombie state." Poetic license or big lie?

Sometimes the distortions are the fault not of the filmmaker but of the writer whose work they adapt. Kesey, who would have known what ECT really was like from his work in the early 1960s as a nurse's aide at the Menlo Park VA Hospital, laid out in words many of the fanciful images in Forman's film version of *Cuckoo's Nest*. Other times errors are in the eyes of the filmgoer. The 2001 Best Picture Oscar winner *A Beautiful Mind* shows economics genius John Nash suffering violent convulsions when he was hospitalized for paranoid schizophrenia. Most moviegoers probably presumed the seizures were the result of electroshock, since it was confusing, and few remembered the actual form of convulsive therapy he got, the long-defunct insulin coma.

Does it matter whether filmmakers get it right depicting ECT? History says it does. During its halcyon days in the 1940s and 1950s, ECT had no public profile, good or bad, being known mainly to doctors, patients, and their families. The image that eventually took hold came directly from the silver screen, which shaped public attitudes toward electroshock even more than what psychiatrists or antipsychiatry activists said or did. *Cuckoo's Nest,* for one, was watched by nearly everyone on the planet, judging from box-office receipts of more than $100 million in America and close to $200 million worldwide. The Forman film did to shock treatment what Alfred Hitchcock's *Psycho* did to old motels: scared people away. A 1983 survey of workers in Ireland aimed at understanding public attitudes to ECT found that nearly two-thirds of respondents had seen the film—twice as many as read about electroshock in newspapers, magazines, or journals—and by the time they left the theater two-thirds of them were "put off ECT." The same was true from Copenhagen to Cairo, New York to New Delhi. McMurphy and his compatriots hoodwinked even young doctors-to-be. Movies were their most frequent source of information about ECT, at 42.4 percent, followed by 25.4 percent who said they got what they knew from college classes, according to a poll of University of Arkansas medical students published in 2001.

Even more affected by what they see on the screen are psychiatric patients. To them, ECT is not an abstraction but an option, one they are less likely to use if a moviemaker as convincing as Milos Forman casts it as torture. Dr. Y. Pritham Raj saw that effect in one of his patients at Duke University who had seen *The Snake Pit* and identified with Virginia Cunningham, the heroine who had a psychotic break and was given ECT. "Before treatment could begin" with his patient, writes Raj, "her misconceptions about hospitals, created by this film, had to be dispelled. This took considerable time and affected the length of her stay." The same thing happened with several patients who said they no longer trusted psychiatrists after watching *A Beautiful Mind*. That 2001 Oscar winner, Raj says, has "introduced a new generation of moviegoers to shock therapy much as *One Flew Over the Cuckoo's Nest* did in 1975, with damaging results."

Movies are not the only way popular culture has defined public attitudes on electroshock. Musicians have zeroed in on the treatment, generally to lance it. Lou Reed did that in his 1974 song "Kill Your Sons," supposedly written in response to electroshock the rock star got as a teenager. "All your two-bit psychiatrists / Are giving you electroshock . . . Don't you know they're gonna kill your sons / Don't you know gonna kill, kill your sons." Newspaper and magazine stories have had a still bigger impact. Most reporters try to be balanced, but they, their editors, and their readers understandably are drawn more to horror stories than to evidence that shock's benefits outweigh its risks. Books, both fiction and nonfiction, are less constrained by standards of fairness. The most gripping and persuasive have included testimonies by people who had ECT, and most of those in the 1960s, 1970s, and 1980s were tales of woe.

"I had been subjected to electric shock treatments that deadened my brain, stole chunks of time from my memory, and left me feeling brutalized," film star Gene Tierney wrote in her 1979 autobiography. "Over the next eight months I underwent nineteen more electric shock treatments, a grand total, I think, of thirty-two. Pieces of my life just disappeared. A mental patient once said it must have been what Eve felt, having been created full grown out of somebody's rib, born without a history. That is exactly how I felt."

Janet Frame and Sylvia Plath, poetesses separated by a generation and a world, told their own remarkably similar horror stories about ECT in their memoirs and in film adaptations of them. "Then something bent down and took hold of me and shook me like the end of the world. Whee-ee-ee-ee-ee, it shrilled, through an air crackling with blue light, and with each flash a great jolt drubbed me till I thought my bones would break and the sap fly out of me like a split plant. I wondered what terrible thing I had done," narrator Esther Greenwood says in Plath's largely autobiographical 1963 novel *The Bell Jar*, apparently echoing Plath's own experience with ECT in her native Massachusetts. Frame got hers in New Zealand. That is where she grew up and in 1985 published the last of a three-volume autobiography which, five years later, was made into the award-winning film *An Angel at My Table*. "I was given the new electric treatment, and suddenly my life was thrown out of focus. I could not remember. I was terrified," Frame wrote. "Electric shock treatment may turn many grim memories out of house and home; what is certain is that it invites as permanent tenants the grim memories of itself, of receiving shock treatment."

The most legendary testimony against electroshock came from America's most legendary writer, Ernest Hemingway. In 1960 and 1961, Hemingway received several series of treatments at the Mayo Clinic to help with his severe depression, paranoia, obsessions, and delusions. Instead, he said, the ECT destroyed his memory. "What is the sense of ruining my head and erasing my memory, which is my capital, and putting me out of business?" Hemingway asked his friend and biographer A. E. Hotchner. "It was a brilliant cure but we lost the patient."

Hemingway finally convinced his Mayo doctors to stop giving him ECT in the spring of 1961. At the end of June he checked out of the clinic and went home to Idaho with his wife, Mary. On the morning of July 2 he got up early, went downstairs dressed in pajamas and robe, and retrieved a twelve-gauge shotgun and box of shells from a closet in the basement. He put the barrel into his mouth, then pulled the trigger. Mary, who had been sleeping upstairs, found him in the sitting room— a "crumpled heap of bathrobe and blood."

Was there a cause and effect between the ECT and his suicide? ECT critics think so, and have drawn the link repeatedly in books, articles, and pamphlets, using it as Exhibit A for just how dangerous it is to shock the brain. James Nagel, former president of the Hemingway Society, also sensed a connection, telling CNN in 1999 that "it was on the first day he returned from his thirty-sixth shock treatment that he killed himself." (In fact, his shock treatments had ceased at least a week before his death and perhaps as much as a month.) Hemingway biographer Jeffrey Meyers offers a mixed picture. ECT clearly made Hemingway's mental illness worse. But Meyers also makes clear that Hemingway had been talking about suicide for half a century, and that near the end of his life he had even more reason to do it given his long list of ailments including impotence, a disfiguring skin condition, alcoholism, diabetes, high blood pressure, and liver disease.

Hotchner, who was Hemingway's confidant as well as his chronicler and is repeatedly quoted by ECT critics, cautions that it is dangerous to blame his suicide on electroshock or any single cause. "The big problem was that instead of being given a complete series of shocks he was given half of them. That left him in a more disturbed state," Hotchner says. "The treatments certainly didn't do him any good, and may have worsened his condition somewhat, but I really think that without shock treatment he would have committed suicide anyway."

∽◯

The early 1980s were the nadir. ECT, which was still a first-line treatment when Hemingway got his in the early 1960s, was distrusted if not despised just twenty years later. The pendulum had swung back as far as it could. A patient who presented with the kind of debilitating depression that ECT could relieve was half as likely to get it in 1980 as a decade before. A medical student who decided on a career in psychiatry was substantially less likely to be schooled in or even told about electroshock. An academic psychiatrist who had been conducting ECT experiments was likely to have been seduced away by pharmaceuticals, where there was more money and less controversy.

Ranking the reasons for that decline is tricky; there were so many and they were so interwoven. Any treatment involving electricity and the brain is bound to be controversial. ECT doctors failed to appreciate that vulnerability, to temper their excesses, and to acknowledge side effects like memory loss. Critics did grasp all that, and effectively cast ECT as a symbol of all that was wrong with big government, bad corporations, and an arrogant medical establishment. The whole debate might have remained underground but for the filmmakers and writers, who recognized a brilliant story even if they did not always discern the difference between fact and fiction. And patients, who in another era might have looked beyond the horror stories, simply switched to Prozac, Zoloft, or one of the other new psychopharmaceuticals.

The results are there to gauge: While some 300,000 people a year were receiving ECT in the early 1960s, twenty years later there were only 60,000. If he had a sense of perspective and whimsy, one of the rare ECT doctors still practicing in 1980 might have paraphrased Hemingway: It was a brilliant cure but we lost the cure.

Seven

LIFTING THE CLOUD

Next thing I know I am waking up. I am back on an upper floor of Massachusetts General Hospital, in the unit where I slept last night. I feel light-headed, groggy, the way you do when anesthesia is wearing off and you are floating in the abyss between sleep and wakefulness. I vaguely recall the anesthesiologist having had me count to ten, but I never got beyond three or four. I remember Charlie Welch and his ECT team, but am not sure I got the treatment. One clue is a slight headache, which they told me ECT might cause but which could have come from the anesthesia. Another is the goo on my hair, where they must have attached the electrodes.

There is one more sign that I did in fact have my first session of seizure therapy: I feel good—I feel alive.

Michael is standing there next to the nurse as I struggle to keep my eyes open, and I give him a big grin. That surprises him right away. After a bit more dozing I am awake for good, and get dressed. Michael takes me to the car, which is in the garage attached to the hospital. I have been warned not to expect too much from any single ECT treatment, especially my first, when doctors are adjusting the dose and fine-tuning their technique to my body and mind. But I already can detect a difference. Feeling this good is truly amazing given where I am coming from, which is a very dark place that has lasted a very long time. Just last night I was so shaky I didn't trust myself to stay in my own house, so I checked in here at Mass. General. That seems like ages ago. As we head home to Brookline, I remember that it is our anniversary. Our thirty-eighth. I turn to Michael and say, "Let's go out for dinner tonight!" He asks, "What?" I say, "I'm serious. Let's do it!"

Michael and I did eat out at a restaurant that night, making an anniversary I wanted to forget into one I will remember always. I was back at the hospital on an outpatient basis the next two weeks for four more treatments. After the second one I went to the hairdresser, then a dinner party, and watched the Red Sox on TV. Over the following four years I have returned to Mass. General and Charlie seven more times.

It is not an exaggeration to say that electroconvulsive therapy has opened a new reality for me. I used to deny when a depressive episode was coming on, to myself and others. I knew how much it would hurt, how long the darkness would last. I just couldn't face it. I thought if I ignored it, it might go away on its own. Now I know there is something that will work and work quickly. It takes away the anticipation and the fear. I call Charlie as soon as I spot the gathering clouds. I also used to be unable to shake the dread even when I was feeling good, because I knew the bad feelings would return, the way they always did after eight months. ECT has wiped away that foreboding. It has given me a sense of control, of hope.

As important, ECT has gotten me off antidepressants. I withdrew slowly, with help from my doctors. Since I have been off I know the full range of my feelings. I get into the car now and put on music, the classical station. I sometimes cry because it conjures up feelings of my dad, who died on March 29, 2003. When I was a child I cried often enough and hard enough that my parents used to say, "Go get the bucket for Kitty's tears." Once I went on antidepressants I couldn't bring myself to tears, whether I was listening to music or mourning my father. The drugs somehow blocked my emotions. Once I went off I was able to read the thousand or so letters we got from people who knew and loved Dad, who had worked with him or considered themselves part of our family. I finally could grieve. I could cry. ECT let me do that. As Michael says, "You can feel your feelings again."

The side effects of antidepressants didn't stop there. They created intestinal issues for me, bowel problems. They made my mouth dry and sex more difficult. I slept more than I should have. None of those complications threatened my life, but each made it less enjoyable. All those things cleared up when I stopped taking the drugs, and it has made a huge difference to me and to my loving husband.

Speed of response is another area where ECT has made a difference. It works right away. I feel the depression beginning to lift after just one treatment, and it is gone entirely within a week to ten days. With antidepressants the effects were gradual. It took time for them to feed into my system. Sometimes it was three weeks or a month before I felt the full power of a particular medication, and even then none of the drugs worked as advertised. With ECT the effect is immediate and as powerful as promised. That's not to say I am not tired after electroconvulsive therapy. I'm not going to run the Boston Marathon, not that I ever could. But the difference between the two treatments is dramatic.

Electroconvulsive therapy has even helped with talk therapy, strange as that may sound. I had been with Roger Weiss, my therapist, for five or six years. After ECT, I was able to work on issues that I couldn't before, with him and on my own. I stopped smoking fifteen months ago and feel terrific about that. I am working on my road rage, which is especially challenging every winter when we head to L.A. and start driving those confounding freeways. I am trying to stop or at least streamline my impulsive shopping and to curb my compulsion for candy and other sweets. I am even addressing what my kids call my sense of entitlement. They kid me for behaving like the "queen bee." It is not ECT per se that is curing me of those bad habits. It is staying well enough for long enough that I can start looking at behaviors I want to change. Why, for instance, do I always introduce myself by my last name as well as first? Kara, Andrea, and John say I am seeking the recognition that comes with the name Dukakis. Whether they are right or not, it was impossible to acknowledge they might be when I was depressed. I wasn't thinking clearly. ECT unfogs your head enough to face issues more honestly.

It isn't just me who sees these differences. Corky, my support group sponsor, calls the effect it has had on me "fabulous," adding that "without ECT I think you eventually might have done away with your life, maybe not on purpose, but through drinking or something. I don't think you would have had four years of sobriety without ECT." After my treatments my dad used to tell Michael, "The other Kitty is back. The good Kitty." Wilma Greenfield, a friend since we were both thirteen, says she, too, despaired that when I was depressed everything about me seemed dulled down. "The new image—the post-ECT one," she says, "is the Kitty I knew when we were growing up together. You return to that very upbeat, very positive person. The sparkle is there. There are no dips."

The kids are more skeptical, having seen me go up, then dip down, with earlier treatments. But John still concludes that ECT has "made a huge difference." Kara says, "I definitely buy into the idea that it's working, at least for now." Andrea worries every time I get ECT that that might be the time when it won't work, but so far those fears have not been borne out.

Michael is less reticent. He knows how self-destructive I was, and how nothing else seemed to help. ECT, he says, is our miracle.

That does not mean I look forward to the treatments. Who would? No one wants electricity shot into their brain, or even to get anesthesia. But when I lie down I know that within seconds I'll be asleep—and that this process is going to make me better. I also know that, like many patients today, I can go home after each treatment rather than stay overnight in the hospital, which makes an enormous difference. That first treatment on our wedding anniversary set the pattern. It lifted the shade on my dark mood. I can be a basket case, but the first ECT always brings me out of that. The next one helps a little more, and the several after that. By the time I was finished with that first series of five, I was myself again.

I have had seven more sets of ECT at Mass. General since the first in 2001, and one at Cedars-Sinai Medical Center in Los Angeles. Some things are the same each time. I stop eating or drinking at midnight the night before, same as I would for any surgery. I am always the first patient in the morning, at seven o'clock, which Dr. Welch arranges to protect my privacy. I always start out at Phillips House, a VIP area in the hospital where I am unlikely to run into other patients and nothing gets put in my regular hospital record. I change out of street clothes into hospital pajamas, then head down in the elevator with Dr. Welch or his associate to the treatment room. I always end up back in that private room in Phillips House where I can fully wake up. I am grateful. Friends who have had ECT tell me they hated waking up in a cubicle with eight or ten patients in different cubicles around them.

Hearing noises, they say, is very frightening. Your memory is shaky at that stage, and the last thing you want is anything unfamiliar, anything that might be scary.

One last thing about my experience with ECT: I am never nervous. The minute I lie down on that table the anxiety is just not there, period. It's not part of my thinking. I know I am going to start feeling better almost right away. I actually wake up hungry, and after a short nap in the hospital I can't wait to get home and have breakfast. Knowing all that helps me get prepared. I have absolute confidence in the team at Mass. General and in the procedure.

Before they begin, Charlie and his colleagues take a series of medical precautions, some of which are particular to me. I get beta-blockers to ensure there is no spike in my blood pressure or cardiac rate. They have raised my dosage of anesthesia because in the early treatments I was waking up a bit early. I get a dose of analgesic to prevent me from getting stiff, which is a special risk since I had serious neck surgery nearly twenty years ago. They wait until I am falling asleep to apply the oxygen mask, because when they did it while I was awake, it dredged up scary memories of the tonsillectomy I had in my own home as a young child. For a while I was getting a tranquilizer because I had some problems with anxiety.

All my treatments have been unilateral, which means the electrodes go on just one side of my head in positions that Charlie says are aimed at minimizing memory loss. The same concern led them to gradually lower the intensity of the stimulus they give me, to a level the doctors say is one-tenth of what Stelian Dukakis probably got in the 1950s. Charlie also has adjusted the waveform of the current to one he says is less vigorous but still strong enough to work for me.

I generally need treatment every seven or eight months, which has always been my timeline for depression returning. It was a full fourteen months between my first and second sets of ECT, which felt great. Several times I have needed another round after just two or three months. Charlie says that is because he and I were experimenting to see whether we could get away with fewer than the normal seven treatments per series, or at least space them farther apart. He also was testing just how low-intensity he could go to minimize the chance of side effects while preserving the ECT's effectiveness. My last set was in April–May of 2005, seven and a half months after the previous one, and I have been doing great since then.

One strange effect that ECT has had on me is to leave me a little hyper. My sister notices how quickly I go back to shopping and spending money on clothing and other things. I can hear Jinny say, "Are you sure you need that?" The answer, of course, is "No, but I want it," a response that alarms my parsimonious spouse. I'm somewhat embarrassed by my free-spending ways and am working on staying away from stores, at least in the aftermath of my treatments. Roger, my therapist, says ECT can actually induce a mild mania, and that it appears to do that with me the same way antidepressants did. Maybe it is just revealing my bipolar personality, with mania naturally following the depression. Whatever it is, the mania is better than the despair and doesn't last long or create real problems. Andrea notices that I call her and my other kids at least once a day after ECT brings me out of depressions—and she says they have a hard time getting me off the phone. I want to know everything they are doing, and all about my six grandkids. Speaking of the grandkids, I love being with them more than anything, but can't really be when I am deep in a depression. ECT lets me get back to myself quicker than before, and get back with my grandchildren.

A nun who contacted me after a story on my ECT appeared

in the *Boston Globe* described how afraid she had been to have ECT. She said, "This is the way I would feel going in for a root canal." As for me, I hate fillings, and don't like to go to the dentist, period. I happened to have had a root canal not long before my first electroconvulsive therapy. In some ways ECT is less traumatic for me than going to the dentist, and certainly less frightening than the root canal. Lots of doctors say I am crazy for thinking something like that, but I don't have negative thoughts about the treatment.

Eight

BODY OF EVIDENCE

*D*r. Stephen Dinwiddie should have hated ECT. His dad was a psychologist, with that profession's bias toward talk therapy and against trying to shock patients out of their anguish. Steve was trained in the 1980s, an era when shock doctors were likened to Spanish inquisitors and ECT was the bête noire of film and books. The young psychiatrist not only enjoyed the movie *One Flew Over the Cuckoo's Nest* enough to see it twice, he agreed with its premise that patients have too little clout and organized psychiatry has more than it merits.

Dinwiddie was drawn to electroshock for a single reason: It helped when no other treatment did, not even wonder drugs.

"At Washington University, where I trained, ECT never really had fallen out of favor, so I got a very good basis for practicing during my four years of residency," explains Dinwiddie, who now runs the ECT program and teaches at the University of Chicago. "I can still quite vividly recall the utter agony I witnessed the first time I admitted a patient with a severe agitated depression. I couldn't then, and can't now, understand how one can allow that sort of experience to go on a moment longer than absolutely necessary. That doesn't mean jumping to ECT immediately, of course. But it does mean instituting some kind of effective treatment quickly and vigorously. Over my first few months in psychiatry I saw how ECT could help people who did not respond to anything else.

"There is an element of selfishness to this, I suppose. It feels pretty good to be able to so quickly help someone. That is, after all, one of the great emotional payoffs of medicine. That isn't to say that ECT is either a panacea or without flaws—but when used in the right way for the right purposes it's of great benefit, and condemning it because it isn't perfect would lead to more suffering and harm, not less."

June Judge was on a similar quest twenty-five years ago for anything that would stem the suffering. Her son Steve had been lying in bed for two months at the Air Force Academy in Colorado Springs, where he was a student. He had lost touch with reality, trying to hang his coat on a light switch and never knowing just where he was. He could not sleep. He would not talk. He had stopped eating, dropping from 204 pounds to 145. His doctors inserted a feeding tube and started him on Haldol. His mother was convinced that he was starving to death and that the drugs were not helping. The prognosis was grim. Judge knew about ECT because her father had gotten it, and it had helped, when he came back from World War II with a catatonia not unlike Steve's. Staff at Steve's military hospital agreed that ECT could help him, but Colorado was a hotbed of the anti-ECT fever engulfing the United States, and Steve could not get treatment there.

"We got him out of there," June remembers, and transferred him to a hospital in Iowa where he received a round of shock treatments. His mother watched the first session. "Within fifteen minutes he was awake and talking to me. It was the first time he had talked to me in two months. They gave him a series of eleven treatments, and he was walking and eating and wanting to go back to school." Steve relapsed three months later, was institutionalized, and finally found a drug treatment that worked. But it was ECT that "allowed him to get back on his feet," June says. "I really think it saved my son's life, and my father's."

As for the attacks that sent the treatment into a tailspin and made it nearly impossible for Steve to get it in Colorado, June is frustrated. "The general public doesn't think anything of pacemakers for the heart," she says. "But pacemakers for the brain—ECT—taps into a primitive fear and stigma."

At a moment when ECT seemed on the verge of disappearing— when academic psychiatrists had become enchanted with miracle medications and organized medicine was embarrassed by shock therapy—it was doctors like Dinwiddie and family members like Judge who rescued it. Neither had a political agenda. They were not attracted by the treatment's glamour—it had none. The choice of ECT was one they backed into because the other options were few and uninviting. Whatever the ballyhoo about psychopharmaceuticals, they did not help Judge's son or many of Dinwiddie's patients. Nothing else did, either.

ECT may have started as a last resort for them, as for others, but the more they saw the more they were drawn in. The treatment was slowly being reinvented in a handful of academic laboratories and psychiatric hospitals. There had always been scientific studies, but early ones generally looked back after the fact and made crude observations of effects and side effects. The new findings drew on state-of-the-art techniques of animal analysis and human trials. A broader set of questions was being explored on how ECT could root out mental illness without rooting out memories. Just as the trifecta of anesthesia, muscle relaxant, and oxygen had helped overcome the treatment's bone-breaking image in the 1950s, so thirty years later electroshock was crossing an equally momentous threshold of scientific precision that made it more attractive for doctors like Dinwiddie to give and patients like Steve Judge to get.

The pendulum on this improbable therapy had swung again. ECT had survived the excesses of its golden age in the 1940s, '50s, and '60s, when it was used on too many patients who did not want it for too many conditions where its impact was doubtful. It hung on through the dark days of the 1970s and early '80s, when few patients or doctors were interested and an army of detractors hoped to administer last rites. Starting around 1985, ECT began a quiet and startling comeback that continues today and is based on a more accurate understanding of just whom it can help.

ECT, says Judge, "is a last resort for people who are starving to death."

∞

Electroshock works best with the mental illness that is most pandemic: depression. Scientists have been studying that treatment-response relationship for more than sixty years. At first they took rough measurements of whether ECT seemed to help depressed patients. Later they carefully compared it to the effect of antidepressant drugs. Other tests contrasted real shock therapy with what researchers call a placebo, or empty pill, and against "sham ECT," where electrodes are hooked up and a subject is put to sleep thinking she is getting electroshock but no current is delivered or seizure induced.*

ECT came out the winner in each case. That was the conclusion of a 1985 report by researchers at the Illinois State Psychiatric Institute, who reviewed the best studies done on ECT. It proved 41 percent more successful in treating depression than a placebo, and 32 percent more than sham ECT. Patients getting electroshock had a 20 percent better chance of improving than those getting tricyclic antidepressants like imipramine

---

*"Sham" studies were run to answer critics who said that ECT works not because of the electricity or seizure, but due to the anesthesia, muscle relaxant, or maybe psychological factors like being in a therapeutic environment or fearing the shock. By giving a comparison group of patients everything but the current and convulsion, researchers were able to refute those arguments.

and amitriptyline, and 45 percent better than with monoamine oxidase inhibitors like Nardil and Parnate.* While the 1985 analysis did not compare ECT against the newer, more widely used antidepressants called selective serotonin reuptake inhibitors (SSRIs), a 1997 study in Germany did, in patients who were resistant to other medications. It found ECT "clearly superior to" and "substantially faster" than Paxil, one of the most effective of the SSRIs.

That does not mean electroshock can help all 19 million Americans said to suffer from depression or that it is equally effective for everyone lumped under that catchall category. Paradoxically, the more complicated the depression, the better ECT works. That is true for people who are psychotically depressed to the point where they have lost touch with reality. It also is true for people whose depression has rendered them unable to move, speak, or even grimace, earning them the diagnosis of catatonia. Such patients need a response quicker than drugs can offer, and ECT often proves life-saving. Other symptoms that predict a good response are loss of appetite, impaired concentration, and lack of interest in socializing, traveling, and other activities that used to provide pleasure. Time is an even better predictor: The more recent the episode of depression, the easier it is for ECT to help. Patients whose depression grows out of preexisting psychiatric or medical troubles generally do less well, unless that trouble was a stroke.

So how well does ECT work for its target population of severely depressed patients? It can offer immediate relief to three-quarters of them, provided it is properly administered. That is a better track record than for any competing treatment, including the prodigal pharmaceuticals that

---

*Comparisons like these are subject to flaws and open to criticism, including that early drug trials used too small a dose over too short a time. But ECT also was often used under less than ideal conditions, and more recent, better-run studies comparing drugs to ECT show similar trends in favor of electroshock.

helped turn doctors and patients away from electroshock during the 1960s and 1970s. There are several critical caveats, however. ECT does not always relieve all symptoms of depression, although it does generally leave patients feeling more vital, able to function socially, and healthier physically as well as emotionally. And it is not a cure; most patients will see their depression come back within months, requiring further treatment with drugs, ECT, talk therapy, or some combination of the three. Yet in the same way that antibiotics reduce the severity of bacterial pneumonia without eliminating the underlying illness, so ECT can offer a break from a debilitating mental disease and a chance to work on a longer-lasting therapy.

"No controlled study has shown any other treatment to have superior efficacy to ECT in the treatment of depression," the surgeon general wrote in his 1999 report on mental health in America. The National Institutes of Health agreed, adding that, with delusional depression, ECT "is superior to either antidepressants or neuroleptics [a tranquilizer often used to treat mental disorders] used alone and is at least as effective as the combination of antidepressants and neuroleptics." Dr. Richard Glass goes a step further in a 2001 editorial in the prestigious *Journal of the American Medical Association,* where he is a deputy editor. "All considerations about ECT must include recognition of the suffering and devastating consequences caused by major depression, a disease with a mortality rate as high as 15 percent," Glass writes. "The results of ECT in treating severe depression are among the most positive treatment effects in all of medicine."

Eileen D. White was the sort of patient Glass must have had in mind when he wrote his editorial. The forty-six-year-old from Sturgis, South Dakota, says she "can't remember a time I wasn't depressed, starting as a teenager." It ruined her career in the air force, preventing her from getting top-secret clearance. She couldn't coax herself out of bed, take a shower, or brush her teeth or her hair. She was hospitalized twelve times during the 1990s. She tried Prozac on four separate occasions, without success.

She tried Depakote, Wellbutrin, and Tegretol. No luck. She was married three times before she was twenty-five, but got divorced each time because "my husbands couldn't live with someone who went through such depressions and would stay in bed literally for weeks. I wrote letters to my parents, my husband, and my doctor explaining that I would probably be much happier being dead. I couldn't take the misery any more of living. I never had any time free of my symptoms."

Finally, in 1999, two days after graduating from a college that took her twelve years to get through, she tried ECT for the first time. The treatment took away memories—of her graduation, the telephone number her parents had had for forty years, even where she kept her spoons. But it gave her back her life. "For the first time in my life I had depression-free moments. I had been anorexic before; I started eating better and gained weight. I was sleeping regularly for the first time in years. My anti-depressants kicked in and started working. It straightened out my brain chemistry," says White, who now speaks across the country about mental illness and recovery. "Since then I have not had one of the depressions where I was bedridden for a week. I love my life right now.

"Although I do have a noticeable difference in my short-term memory, I would have it [ECT] again in an instant. I lost about a month to the ECT, but I gained a new and wonderful life."

White's therapists are even more bullish about her recovery. "After her third ECT treatment she suddenly was sitting upright in the chair in my office. She was able to look at me and make good eye contact in a way she hadn't before. Her whole expression just seemed like a veil had been lifted," recalls Frederick Magnavito, the psychologist who treated her at the Veteran's Hospital in Fort Meade, South Dakota. "ECT laid a great foundation for what she accomplished." Dr. Thomas Jewitt is the psychiatrist who referred White for ECT and who now provides her with psychotherapy and drugs. "Eileen was hard work, let me tell you," he says. "She was basically completely and totally disabled, but for some reason I had a conviction there was somebody there. Now look at what she is. She has emerged from the flames. Not everyone is like this. She had a very innate capability, but who knew? It has been pretty incredible—kind of scary."

Thomas Fitzgerald knows more about electricity than Eileen White and most other fellow ECT patients, but that knowledge was not reassuring. "I got belted by electricity a couple times at work, which makes you respect it a lot," says the sixty-one-year-old electrician from Methuen, Massachusetts. That respect, combined with images of Randall Patrick McMurphy getting shocked in *Cuckoo's Nest,* gave Fitzgerald pause when his doctor recommended two years ago that he try ECT. He had been on medications, but they had lost their power to fend off the depression he suffered for twenty years. The electroshock worked well enough that Fitzgerald continues to get a maintenance treatment every six weeks. "I haven't been depressed for two years," he reports. "All's I know is I feel good. If I have to do ECT the rest of my life, if that's the price I have to pay, I'll keep doing it."

That a jolt to the head can lift Fitzgerald out of his despair and lethargy is surprising enough. But it is truly counterintuitive that ECT works equally well for depression's mirror image: the grandiosity and hyperactivity of mania. Sometimes mania appears by itself. Other times it alternates with bouts of depression and is called bipolar disorder, an illness that afflicts more than 2 million Americans but often goes undiagnosed because the highs are dismissed as natural euphoria. ECT can be effective with either form of mania.

Electroshock's potential in treating mania should have been apparent from the very beginning, when Ugo Cerletti treated his first patient in 1938. Although everyone at the time thought S.E. suffered just from schizophrenia, Cerletti later confided his suspicion that the engineer from Milan also was manic. ECT quickly became the standard treatment for mania and what was then called manic depression, and it continued to be widely used until the drug revolution of the late 1950s. It was displaced first by Thorazine, then by lithium, and more recently by anticonvulsant medications like Depakote that are often combined with lithium. Yet in a 1988 study comparing ECT head-to-head with lithium, electroshock worked faster, confirming earlier reviews and the experience of practitioners over the decades. ECT is used today in mania cases where the delirium is striking, mood elevations are stubborn, and one drug after another does nothing.

Andy Behrman is one of those cases. "Manic depression for me is like having the most perfect prescription eyeglasses with which to see the world," Behrman writes in his 2002 memoir *Electroboy*, which was an ECT nurse's nickname for him. "Everything is precisely outlined. Colors are cartoonlike, and, for that matter, people are cartoon characters. Sounds are crystal clear, and life appears in front of you on an oversized movie screen. I suppose that would make me the director of my own insanity, but I can only wish for that kind of control. In truth, I am removed from reality and have no direct way to connect to it. My actions are random—based on delusional thinking, warped intuition, and animal instinct. When I'm manic, my senses are so heightened, I'm so awake and alert, that my eyelashes fluttering on the pillow sound like thunder."

Behrman ran through thirty-seven different drugs trying to battle his mania, then turned to the only alternative, shock. While he is not a fan of the treatment because of the memory loss and other side effects he suffered, Behrman says that "ECT is a great choice for people who come to the end of the line and are just totally unsuccessful with medications."

Paul Cumming says that before getting ECT in 2001 he was taking high doses of as many as seven drugs to treat his bipolar disorder; afterward he has done well on low doses of two or three medications. His four sessions of electroshock, he adds, gave him "five years of stability and counting, the longest stretch I've had." Cumming, who lives in the mountain town of Descanso near San Diego and works for an Internet-based mental health network, knows that ECT has a "horrific reputation" and "the thought of it scares people." But it never frightened him. Quite the opposite. He was so enthusiastic that "I actually tried to do ECT on myself in 1992. I bought a cranial unit that has been popular since the 1980s for helping with muscle pain. It gave tiny, tiny bits of pulsing electricity. I didn't realize that ECT is a seizure therapy, not an electrical therapy."

Steve L. came to ECT with the same sense of desperation as Cumming and Behrman, but left without the same satisfaction. His bipolar diagnosis dates to 1969, and often left him feeling "like a Stepford wife who didn't have even a painted smile on my face. I was an exhibition of a living death." He was on as many as thirty medications, with varying degrees and durations of success, but in 1997 he was desperate enough that his doctor suggested ECT. "I went in defeated," the writer and public speaker from outside Boston recalls, "thinking that I must be incredibly pathetic because I had to have ECT." After fourteen treatments he realized that even this last-resort therapy was not working: "It did not help me at all." ECT may deliver for 75 percent of depressed and bipolar patients, but that leaves 25 percent empty-handed, including Steve. Still, he stops short of warning others off: "I would never say to someone, 'You should not use ECT.' I have known too many people who responded markedly well to it. I just happen not to be one of those. . . . One man's treasure might be another man's trash. ECT might be a lifesaver for someone else."

If it is illogical that ECT works equally well with mania and depression, it is even more puzzling that a treatment premised on inducing seizures should aid in controlling seizures. But ECT does, helping treat epilepsy along with the debilitating depression that often accompanies it. That mechanism has fascinated researchers since the 1940s. It involves ECT setting off an anticonvulsant reaction in the brain that limits the duration of the very seizure it is inducing. Just how that happens is unclear, but there is considerable evidence that it works, beginning with the way the amount of electricity needed to induce a seizure often rises over the course of ECT treatments. More compelling proof comes from the observation that ECT can actually stop seizures in animals, and in man.

It was a three-year-old child who in 1941 offered one of the first successful tests of electroshock as an anticonvulsant therapy. Five years later there was sufficient evidence for Lothar Kalinowsky to write, "In patients having spontaneous convulsions at regular intervals, an artificial convulsion offered some protection against a spontaneous fit which, occurring under uncontrolled conditions, might endanger the patient and jeopardize his social condition." ECT critics debunk that notion, saying that shock therapy is much more likely to cause rather than control epilepsy. But researchers in New York and South Carolina have had positive results in patients with stubborn epilepsy, including children. Those findings are especially resonant considering how common depression is among people with epilepsy, who commit suicide at a rate nearly ten times that of the general population. Britain's Royal College of Psychiatrists feels sufficiently comfortable with ECT's antiepileptic properties to recommend it as a treatment when anticonvulsant drugs do not work.

Nancy Kopans's brother Gary was not an epileptic, but he did experience an epilepticlike seizure. It happened after the death of his mother in 1988, when he was depressed to the point of "being trapped in a personal hell." Gary is mentally retarded, and because of his depression he had been relocated from a group home to a psychiatric hospital in New York. Doctors put him on a variety of medications; none worked. What did work was the spontaneous seizure that, as his sister recalls, "shocked him back to being the happy person he was, wide-eyed, gregarious. We went ice skating in the middle of this, he went around and around the rink." The improvement did not last long, but it did give his physicians the idea that "something might be going on here with electrical currents.

"His doctors explained to us that a person of normal or high intelligence can often lift himself out of depression. But Gary was just stuck, he could not hoist himself out of the trough. They told us about this new treatment. They said it still was experimental but it no longer was like *One Flew Over the Cuckoo's Nest*," recalls Nancy, who along with her sister Lauren is Gary's guardian. "He probably had two to three treatments and it worked. He didn't sink back."

The medical literature is rife with reports of ECT being used on patients like Gary, with mental retardation along with psychiatric disorders. A 2001 study by researchers in the Netherlands pored through all the research and found that, of forty-four such patients, "ECT was effective and without important side effects" in thirty-seven, a success rate of 84 percent. The remaining seven patients did not improve or suffered severe agitation or other side effects that made doctors stop the treatments. Given how often mental illness accompanies mental retardation, and how effective ECT can be, the authors wondered why it is not used more often. The answer, they wrote, is legal limits like those in Missouri where ECT is not allowed for the retarded, and ethical worries that shock treatment will be used now, the way it was in the past, as punishment or behavioral conditioning.

Parkinson's disease and neuroleptic malignant syndrome are two other medical conditions where ECT is used, sometimes with remarkable effect. In the former, electroshock not only can help with depression accompanying the chronic and progressive ailment but also can ease rigidity and make it easier to move. The relief generally is short-lived—from hours to months—although ongoing ECT treatments can extend those benefits. Likewise, electroshock can relieve the fever, rigidity, and other effects of neuroleptic malignant syndrome, a sometimes-fatal condition that mimics the effects of lethal catatonia. As for obsessions and compulsions, there is little scientific proof of its helping and some that it actually hurts, although there is also half a century of encouraging anecdotal evidence. And obsessive-compulsive disorder—like Parkinson's, mental retardation, Huntington's disease, multiple sclerosis, muscular dystrophy, and central nervous system syphilis—often carries in tow a deep depression that ECT clearly can help relieve.

Doctor and author Sherwin B. Nuland saw that firsthand more than thirty years ago when he was losing the battle against OCD and depression: "I was, in fact, completely disabled by pathological preoccupations and fears," recalls the surgeon, bioethicist, and medical historian. "Obsessions with coincidences; fixations on recurrent numbers; feelings of worthlessness and physical or sexual inadequacy; religious anxieties of guilt and concerns about God's will; ritualistic thinking and behavior— they crowded in on one another so forcefully as to occupy every lacuna of my mind. . . . So profound was my depression and so tyrannical the jumble of unbidden thoughts and compulsive actions that they ruled the hours of my days and the days of my years. I feared the obsessions, I feared the threatening loss of control, and I feared the fear—all at once. Mostly, I feared for my sanity."

Doctors at the psychiatric hospital where Nuland was being treated were so skeptical of his recovering that they scheduled a lobotomy, a procedure long since out of favor. The brain-severing surgery was avoided only because a young resident convinced his senior colleagues to try ECT instead. "At first, the newly instituted treatment made not a whit of difference," Nuland, who teaches at the Yale School of Medicine, writes in his memoir *Lost in America*. "The number of electroshock treatments mounted, but still no improvement took place. The total would eventually reach twenty. Somewhere around the middle of the course, a glimmer of change made itself evident, which encouraged the skeptical staff to continue a series of treatments they had begun only to mollify a promising young man in training. In the beginning only a bit but after a while more palpably, the depression began to lighten and the obsessions became less insistent. As inexplicable as it seems, I sometimes forgot to think about them entirely. I was sleeping until a normal hour each morning, and I would wake thinking clearly and remaining optimistic for most of the day."

❦

Certain populations of patients are substantially more likely to be considered for ECT than others, for good reason.

People thinking about killing themselves top the list. The logic for using ECT as a first-choice treatment with suicidal patients is compelling: They need something faster acting than antidepressants, which can take weeks to kick in. ECT generally starts working within a couple of treatments, meaning a couple of days. The science backing up such early intervention has been murky, at least until recently. Some reports showed that ECT does not prevent suicide; others argued that it reduces overall mortality and suicide in particular. The confusion stems in part from the fact that most early studies failed to ask whether patients who got ECT were sicker than those who did not. A more basic difficulty is the expectation of what ECT can do. Its effect, however positive, is short-lived, and even patients who are temporarily spared from suicide often relapse into depression and try again.* But even a short-lived effect is critical if it saves a patient's life and gives her a chance to find a longer-lasting treatment.

The newest and most exhaustive report on ECT and suicide offers convincing evidence that the therapy does produce a rapid if fleeting reduction in suicidal thinking. That study, published in 2005 and involving 131 depressed patients who said they were actively contemplating killing themselves, found that 38 percent stopped thinking about suicide after just one week of ECT treatment. Seventy-six percent responded after three weeks. Those results are convincing enough that doctors should think about turning to ECT earlier with their most deeply depressed patients, say the authors, whose research is supported by the National In-

---

*For each suicide a patient attempts, the risk of another attempt rises by 30 percent over the two years following discharge from the hospital.

stitute of Mental Health. The current practice of waiting until drugs and other treatments are tried and fail, they add, "unnecessarily puts suicidal psychiatrically ill patients at substantial risk."

Whatever the scientists say, Leslie Sladek-Sobczak knows that ECT saved her life—twice. The first time her antidepressants stopped working she was admitted to the hospital and put on suicide watch. But after her watchers had done their spot check, "I took my shoelaces, tied them around my neck, then took a pen and twisted it until it would twist no more," says Sladek-Sobczak, a mental health worker in Traverse City, Michigan. "Had the doctor not walked by then, I would have strangled myself." After her first round of ECT, the thoughts of suicide subsided and she went back on antidepressants for another five years. Then, without warning, the drugs stopped working again. She was worried about hurting herself, and ECT once more offered a bridge. "It gives you the immediate response you need when you are in the darkest spot there is. You don't have to wait six weeks to find out if it worked or not, the way you do with medications. A lot can happen in six weeks when you are in that darkness."

It is a familiar story, one told by patients who have weathered ECT with few complications and others, like Carolyn, who "couldn't even find my way to the post office I had been going to for thirty years. I could watch every TV rerun during the summer like it was a brand-new show." Precious as those memories were, what matters more to Carolyn is that she is alive. One day nearly ten years ago she was feeling especially hopeless. She was under the spell of a depression so severe that she had stopped eating or showering, was smoking two to three packs of cigarettes a day, and spent her waking hours drinking coffee and staring blankly at the television screen. She had tried endless combinations of medications—"I stopped counting at about twenty-eight"—along with daily talk therapy and periodic hospitalizations. "I just felt like nothing would ever work," she remembers. "I was alone in my apartment and decided I wanted to go to sleep—to go to sleep and not wake up. I took all the medications I could find in my house, it was handfuls, probably a couple months worth of Lamictal, probably a hundred or so Tylenol. My therapist happened to call shortly after I had taken them. I was kind of half-awake, half-asleep. I picked up the phone and I guess she called the police on her other phone. She kept me on the phone until they arrived and brought me to the hospital. I don't know if they pumped my stomach. I do know they gave me charcoal."*

They also gave Carolyn ECT, which she had had once before. "It pulled me up enough out of the hole that I could function to go to my appointments, take my medication daily, and try to work with my doctors. It was one of the most difficult things I have ever done in my life. I have memory problems as a residual of it; however, I'm alive. That was the main point." A second residual is the stigma, what she calls "some kind of freak show," which is why Carolyn, who lives south of Boston, asks that only her first name be used. "Not a whole lot of people in my life know about my ECT," she explains. "If I say I'm taking Prozac that's culturally acceptable. But if I say I'm taking ECT people say, 'Shock treatments!' They think of *One Flew Over the Cuckoo's Nest*. It's hard to say to people how wonderfully it works."

If suicidality is the most compelling reason people turn to ECT, old age is a close second. It is tempting to attribute that to the facts that the elderly are well insured, physically and sometimes mentally frail, and therefore ripe for exploitation. The truth is that older Americans suffer at higher rates precisely the forms of depression where ECT is most likely to be prescribed. They often have heart and other medical conditions that prevent their taking antidepressants. Even when they can take antidepressants, there is a lower success rate than with younger patients. All of which makes the elderly more likely to consider ECT.

---

*Lamictal is an anticonvulsant used to treat bipolar disorder. Charcoal is used on patients who overdose to bind the drugs, keeping them out of the blood until they are expelled in the stool.

ECT, in turn, seems to do a better job of relieving depression in older people than with younger ones. That was the conclusion of a 1999 study involving 268 patients at four hospitals. It found a 54 percent response rate in patients fifty-nine and younger, a 73 percent response in those sixty to seventy-four, and a 67 percent response with "old-old" patients seventy-five and up. The American Psychiatric Association and Britain's Royal College of Psychiatrists agree that ECT works especially well for the elderly—one of the few treatments in medicine where that is the case. Why? Older patients who cannot tolerate drugs get ECT as a first rather than last resort. That lets it go to work before the episode of depression has settled in and is tougher to dislodge. It also means that the group getting ECT is not just those who are drug-resistant and may be harder to treat. There is one more reason that ECT makes special sense the older you are, says the surgeon general: Depression at an advanced age often brings with it an inability to eat or even walk that, if untreated, can be deadly.

ECT use among the young is more problematic. That is partly for fear of harming the still-forming brains of children. It also is a reaction to experiments like the one Lauretta Bender conducted half a century ago at New York's Bellevue Hospital, with patients as young as thirty-four months getting twenty treatments. Her work made clear to psychiatrists that while they might escape notice by giving electroshock to consenting adults, controversy is inevitable when the patients are society's youngest and most helpless. An equivalent caution, born of reason blended with fear, has spilled over into the research world. Studying ECT use among children runs into the same ethical minefield as other experiments involving the young, who cannot give truly informed consent. Recent evidence that children's brains are affected differently by psychotropic drugs, possibly raising the risk of suicide, makes it even more problematic to administer to kids ECT or any treatment that relies on altering brain chemistry. The result is that only a modest number of studies have been done on ECT in children, and most of them reviewed evidence after treatment rather than designing beforehand the controlled trials that offer a clearer test of a treatment's safety and effectiveness.

Yet the studies that have been run suggest that ECT can offer the young, and even the very young, benefits nearly identical to adults. That was the finding of a 1997 review by Australian researchers who scoured sixty reports prepared over the previous half century, involving 396 patients aged eighteen or younger. They found a 63 percent rate of improvement for depression, 80 percent with mania, 42 percent for schizophrenia, and 80 percent with catatonia. "ECT in the young," the authors conclude, "seems similar in effectiveness and side effects to ECT in adults." Those authors and others also talked to kids who had gotten ECT, and their parents, and found widespread acceptance of the procedure. In Paris, 60 percent of young patients and 83 percent of their parents said they would agree to have ECT again if needed. In Australia, 86 percent of parents said they would approve of further sessions for their children if needed, and 79 percent would have ECT themselves.

So why do several states ban ECT use among children by law and even more by practice? And why is electroshock never raised as an option by most child psychiatrists? Those are the kinds of questions the American Academy of Child and Adolescent Psychiatry considered in a multiyear investigation of the treatment. Part of the problem, it concluded in its 2004 report, was "historical misuse" of ECT. It also blamed "inaccurate media portrayal" for unnecessarily alarming the public. Legal limits on ECT have the effect of "potentially denying some individuals effective treatment," the academy advised, adding that "when an appropriate clinical situation does present, the clinician should consider its use."

Alisson Wood is glad her doctor considered it during her freshman year in high school, when she was so depressed she could not get out of bed. Before she turned thirteen she was diagnosed with bipolar type II, which includes at least one episode of major depression and one of a milder mania known as hypomania. By age fifteen, she was bedridden and thinking about killing herself. Her doctor prescribed antidepressants, mood stabilizers, anticonvulsants, sleep aids, and other medications including Neurontin, lithium, Depakote, Ambien, Sonata, Ativan, Thorazine, nortriptyline, Wellbutrin, Prozac, Paxil, Zoloft, Serzone, Pamelor, trazodone, and Effexor. Some made her hallucinate, others caused her hair to fall out. Her parents reluctantly decided she should try ECT. "I had bad jaw pain," recalls Alisson, who is now twenty-one. "I felt as if someone punched me on both sides of my jaw. I had lots of memory loss. I couldn't remember my boyfriend's name. Physically, I didn't react well to it."

While she discontinued the electroshock after eight treatments, she says, "I wasn't as actively suicidal after ECT." And although it took her another year and a half to "get out of bed and accomplish anything in my life," she credits ECT with "giving me that first push. I wish I had done more." ECT, she adds, "is one of mental health's quiet secrets. I think people should definitely know more about it, that it's still out there. It isn't quite like what happened in *One Flew Over the Cuckoo's Nest*. The fact is, it does help a lot of people."

Another group that ECT helps is pregnant women. Pregnancy often brings with it bottomless depression and sky-high mania. It also brings a rightful reluctance to take medications, including antidepressants, for fear of injuring the fetus. Enter ECT, which many psychiatrists consider the treatment of choice during all three trimesters. A 1994 study looked at three hundred reports of ECT use during pregnancy, starting in 1942 and ending in 1991. "Electroconvulsive therapy is a relatively safe and effective treatment during pregnancy" so long as care is taken to monitor the mother and developing child, the study concluded. "In many instances of active mood disorder during pregnancy, the risks of untreated symptoms may outweigh the risks of ECT."

⚭

Nearly seventy years after its launch, researchers also know more about where ECT has a less dramatic effect or none at all.

Schizophrenia is one such condition. It was ECT's first target and remained one of its most popular through the 1940s and 1950s, a time when the frightening diagnosis was applied to almost everyone in the asylum, including many whose actual disease was depression, mania, manic depression, or drug addiction. Thorazine and other antipsychotic drugs started to displace ECT for treating schizophrenics in the 1950s, and the defection picked up steam through the 1960s and 1970s. By the time doctors and patients began to sense the limits and complications of the miracle drugs in the 1980s and afterward, the world of schizophrenia had changed in a way that was unfriendly to ECT. The treatment was no longer offered in many state mental hospitals that housed schizophrenic patients; others with the illness were no longer institutionalized, and some of them no longer had access to electroshock or any other treatment. An even bigger transformation was that ECT had gone from being a first-choice treatment for schizophrenia to a backup, with patients referred today only after antipsychotic and neuroleptic medications have failed. The upshot is that while in 1980 schizophrenia accounted for 16.5 percent of in-hospital ECT usage, by 1986 that number had tumbled to 6.5 percent, and today it almost certainly has slipped further.

Scientists also have been taking a hard look at the use of ECT with schizophrenia and have rendered a judgment kinder than the practitioners. While reports from ECT's earliest days of a 75 percent response rate have not held up with schizophrenia the way they did with depression, more rigorous reviews demonstrate that it can help schizophrenic patients with symptoms known to respond to electroshock, including depression, catatonia, paranoia, and overexcitement. Even when those syndromes are not present ECT can help, just not as often or by as much. One way to raise the odds is to start treatment as close as possible to the onset of the disease generally and the current episode especially. Another is to combine ECT with antischizophrenia drugs like chlozapine. Convulsive therapy is less likely to work with patients who have unwavering, persistent schizophrenia. Yet even there, since drugs seldom work, many psychiatrists say it is worth trying ECT.

Valerie did try. The Kentuckian has a condition called schizoaffective disorder, which combines symptoms of schizophrenia and bipolar disorder. She started getting ECT in 1999, having failed to find relief from a litany of antipsychotic medicines. "The hallucinations went away eight to ten weeks after the ECT, and oh, yes, that was the reason," says the thirty-four-year-old, who asks that her last name not be used. "It was just phenomenal to have ten weeks of silence." The voices eventually came back, but her medications keep them down to what she describes as volume four on a scale of one to ten. "There's a possibility," Valerie adds, "that it was the ECT that made my meds more effective. If anyone asked me for advice, I would say ECT would be very beneficial."

For substance abuse, anxiety and adjustment disorders, and the more persistent but less intense form of depression called dysthymia, advice is clearer-cut on whether or not to get ECT. The answer is no. While ECT can help when secondary and severe depression sets in, it does not treat the underlying disorder and can make neuroses worse. Another rule of thumb is that ECT works with biologically based depressions, not with those based on a death in the family, severed romance, or other changes in circumstance, no matter how life-upending. ECT can pose a risk for people with retinal detachments, certain cerebral lesions, high anesthetic risk, and other heart and brain conditions.

While academic researchers generally concur that ECT is not worth trying with disorders like these, doctors in the community sometimes do not. A 1999 study of ECT use in New England found that 13.5 percent of the time it was used for conditions like dysthymia where there is no evidence it works. That may have been due to the physician's lack of training, or to his consciously deciding that ECT was worth a shot with patients who had run out of options even if their symptoms did not fit the ideal profile. In other cases the problem is failing to utilize ECT often enough when it can help, like with old people who are depressed. The treatment sometimes is terminated sooner than it should be, or performed using outdated techniques or equipment. The result is that in community hospitals, ECT is not nearly as effective as at university medical centers, where patient selection and treatment method are more carefully controlled. The silver lining in such findings is that minor tinkering with technique could radically improve the odds that electroshock will work.

Another factor that lowers ECT's success rate has to do with the kinds of patients who are referred for treatment. By definition they have the most tenacious, hard-to-treat illnesses, since ECT typically is recommended only after someone does not respond to several antidepressants, antipsychotics, or other psychopharmaceuticals. A 1996 study of one hundred patients with depression found that those who did not get better with antidepressants had response rates of just 63.1 percent immediately after treatment with ECT and 47.7 percent a week later, compared to 91 and 74 percent at the same points for patients with no known drug-resistance. Failure to respond to older antidepressants—tricyclic and heterocyclic ones like Tofranil and Adapin—was the best predictor of a poor outcome with ECT. A history of failure with today's most common antidepressants, SSRIs, also forecasts problems with ECT, although not as definitively.

Findings like these send a mixed message to ECT patients. For the almost two-thirds who are resistant to antidepressants, the studies are a discouraging omen of problems with ECT. Yet even with that lowered rate of success, ECT offers their best chance of improving. They already have failed with psychopharmacy, and often with psychotherapy, so electroshock is about all that is left. ECT doctors can sometimes enhance the odds for medication-resistant patients by getting to them sooner after depression sets in and offering them a more intensive treatment program.

The most profound limitation of ECT is that even when it works expeditiously and effectively, the effects typically do not last long. More than half of depressed patients treated with electroshock will experience a return of symptoms within a year, generally within a few months. With medication-resistant patients who respond to ECT, the relapse rate is roughly twice as high, meaning that most if not all can expect the disabling illness to come back soon and with a vengeance. That is probably because the antidepressants other ECT patients use to keep them in remission have shown they do not work for this drug-resistant group. High rates of relapse should not be surprising since major depression, like diabetes and heart disease, is generally a sickness that has to be treated for life. The same way patients helped by antidepressants can expect symptoms to return if the medicines are terminated, so with ECT the effects of treatment often are temporary and symptoms come back when the therapy is stopped.

Understanding why relapse happens does not make it easier for patients to bear, and has had doctors scrambling for responses. It is clear that some sort of ongoing therapy is needed to prolong the short-term benefits of ECT. Drugs are a natural choice, although research and logic argue against using medications that have failed in the past, and argue for combining different drugs rather than relying on one alone. Using lithium together with the antidepressant nortriptyline, for instance, lowered the relapse rate to 39.1 percent in a recent study where patients were followed for six months. That compares to a 60 percent rate for those getting just nortriptyline, and 84 percent among patients getting no post-ECT treatment. The drug combination might have worked even better, the authors speculated, if patients had started on antidepressants during rather than after the course of ECT, or if electric shock therapy had been tapered over a few weeks rather than stopped cold turkey.

Another approach is to continue the patient on ECT for an extra six months, beginning with one session a week and decreasing to about once a month, in the hope of keeping her from plunging back into depression. That strategy seems eminently logical: Why stop ECT if it is working and the patient is tolerating it? Early studies suggest that follow-up ECT often works—not only lowering the rate at which patients relapse into their immediate episode of depression, which typically lasts up to six months, but also preventing them from sinking into new episodes. More rigorous tests are under way with 184 depressed patients at five medical centers across the United States, comparing ongoing ECT with the potent drug combination of nortriptyline and lithium. So far the two are performing practically identically, giving hope that ECT can help keep mental illness at bay for months and even years, and that electroshock given alongside powerful drugs might work better than either independently.

That is no surprise to Dr. Herbert Fox, a Manhattan psychiatrist who has spent years fine-tuning his system of ongoing ECT. He gives an initial series of five to seven treatments to get depressive symptoms under control. Next he administers follow-ups once a week for two to three weeks, then once every two weeks, then once a month. "The ECT treatments," Fox explains, "don't cure the illness but they suppress the symptoms while the episode of depression runs its natural course." How long an episode lasts differs with the individual, and even within individuals depression can resurface with increasing frequency over time. "It's like with a cassette recorder," Fox adds. "Something pushes the start button and the tape has to run through. ECT treatments push down the volume button so you don't hear anything, you don't feel the symptoms."

Christina Heath saw firsthand how ongoing ECT could help, and how knowing when to have it was more art than science. The sixty-four-year-old mental health advocate from Utah had her first treatment in 1995 to help treat a bipolar disorder that had her "living in a fog, living on a different planet. I was really sick." In the beginning she got ECT "on a weekly basis, then less often, with a leveling off at two to three a month. I was determining when I needed an ECT. Whenever I felt like I was having an episode I'd call in and ask for it. . . . ECT gave me my life back, literally."

❧

What gave ECT its life back was a growing realization in the 1980s that the wonder drugs were not wonderful for everyone, and could be dangerous for some. There was also compelling evidence that ECT could help many of those whom drugs could not. That evidence would never have surfaced, or been put into practice, but for the stubbornness of a few psychiatrists who kept ECT alive when their colleagues preferred to give it a quiet burial.

Dr. Max Fink was first and foremost among the revivalists. He watched his first ECT as a medical student in the 1940s and started giving it regularly during his residency in 1952, ECT's heyday. He kept giving it as his colleagues jumped ship. Fink, who trained as a neurologist as well as a psychiatrist and psychoanalyst, in 1979 wrote his generation's definitive primer on ECT, *Convulsive Therapy: Theory and Practice*. It was the first-ever U.S. textbook devoted exclusively to electroshock. He founded and for a decade edited *Convulsive Therapy*, the only scientific journal just on ECT. To Dr. Richard Abrams, Fink's protégé and author of his own popular text on ECT, the contribution by Fink that mattered most came in the late 1950s. "When many of the leading ECT practitioners in this country were purveying their anecdotal and often self-serving claims for one or another particular treatment method," Abrams writes, "Max was conducting and publishing carefully controlled studies on virtually every aspect of ECT: clinical, electrophysiological, pharmacological, neuropsychological, biochemical, psychosocial, and, of course, theoretical. . . . When the parvenu geniuses of psychopharmacology tolled the death-knell of ECT, who but Max (himself a leading psychopharmacologist) was there to remind them that their report of its demise was premature?" Fink, Abrams concludes in a 1994 editorial in *Convulsive Therapy*, "virtually single-handedly nursed ECT back to life while the rest of the psychiatric community looked the other way."

Fink and his compatriots stuck by electroshock partly because they found the new drugs wanting. Antidepressants, antipsychotics, and other pharmaceuticals did help millions deal with symptoms of debilitating mental illness. But they took as long as six weeks to go to work, and their side effects were overwhelming for many. The early antidepressants often brought with them dry mouth, constipation, bladder problems, sexual dysfunction, blurred vision, dizziness and drowsiness, and an elevated heart rate. Newer ones have their own down sides, from headaches and nausea to agitation, insomnia, and, once again, troubles performing sexually. The problems often crossed the line from nuisance to danger for patients who were elderly, physically as well as mentally ill, or pregnant.

For others the issue with psychotropics was not so much their complications as their failure to work at all. An average of one in five patients suffered from such medication resistance. Sometimes the problem was the way the drugs were administered. If prescribed by a state-of-the-art psychopharmacologist, drawing on the range of options and combinations, the failure rate fell to about 10 percent. But in the real world—where treatment was less precise, drugs that once worked petered out over time, and some symptoms inevitably resurfaced—the washout rate could reach 40 percent. When that happened, ECT was there to fill the gap.

The drug revolution was not the only shake-up in the mental health world during the mid-1900s. The move away from the asylum was equally radical, with the number of patients in state and county mental hospitals plummeting from a high of 559,000 in 1955 to just over 100,000 thirty years later. That dramatic remaking of America's mental health system was precipitated by the recognition that the community, rather than the nuthouse of old, is the best place for the mentally ill to get well. It was made possible by the discovery that conditions like schizophrenia and depression have a biological basis and can at least be kept under control by the new generation of medications. And it worked for many, as they found jobs, homes, and lives in the wider community or in the network of halfway houses, overnight shelters, and daytime club-houses quietly erected in neighborhoods across the United States.

But there were holes in the move to community mental health, just as there had been in the boundless embrace of psychiatric drugs. In most states, waiting lists for group homes numbered in the thousands, and still do. A third or more of the homeless are mentally ill, wandering city streets from Boston to Berkeley, convinced they are Christ or Madame Curie. Others are in jails, prisons, or the private psychiatric hospitals and psychiatric wards of general hospitals that took the place of shuttered state and country mental hospitals. While many of those who continue to suffer get no aid at all, some who can afford to turn to private hospitals for the very shock treatment that helped doom the old public asylums.

It was not just defects in the drug and community approaches that fueled ECT's comeback in the 1980s, but electroshock's strengths. The other somatic treatments of the early twentieth century, from insulin coma and Metrazol to sleep therapy and lobotomy, had died, a product of too many side effects or too little effectiveness. ECT, by contrast, proved again and again that it was too valuable to be jettisoned with its sister therapies. It survived because it was needed and it worked. That is why patients continued to get ECT in the new era, when most finally had a voice in what treatment they received, and why a critical mass of doctors kept doing it, despite being branded "shock docs." "It was love at first sight. I saw a couple patients go from being at death's door to full recovery because of ECT and I absolutely fell in love with this process of treating depression," says Dr. Charles Welch, who has run the ECT program at Massachusetts General Hospital since 1980 and since 2001 has been Kitty Dukakis's doctor. "It's sort of like being an obstetrician in that the vast majority of cases have a happy ending."

Today, professors like Harvard University's Welch and the University of Chicago's Dinwiddie are ensuring that psychiatrists-in-training are at least exposed to ECT, and some of those young doctors are referring patients for it or administering it themselves. That does not mean it is easy, as Columbia ECT researcher Harold Sackeim notes, "for people involved with ECT to go home at night and tell their children, 'I'm a shock doctor.' It's not lucrative and doesn't win you fame or fortune. But we're impressed by the outcome, that's why we provide it." It also remains difficult to find a hospital or clinic offering the procedure, but it is easier than it was. More research is being done in the field. More articles are getting published. Practitioners now are so anxious for ways to increase the procedure's effectiveness and diminish its still-considerable side effects that, as Sackeim says, "it is one of the only areas in science where what we concoct through research gets translated almost immediately in the field."

Despite those encouraging developments, ECT today finds itself in an awkward posture: It may be the most effective weapon that psychiatrists have against stubborn mental ailments, but it almost always is reserved as a last resort. The reasons are understandable. They have partly to do with medicine, and the requirement that ECT be delivered in a clinical setting with anesthesia and other intrusive arrangements. The other part is fear of memory loss and related side effects. The result? Some patients suffer longer than they need to before trying electroshock, while others wait so long that it has less chance of working.

That status as a last resort may be changing, albeit slowly. ECT already is a frontline treatment for those whom it has helped before, as well as for certain elderly patients, pregnant women, and others unable to tolerate drugs. New research is beginning to make it easier for psychiatrists to predict which patients are less likely to benefit from drugs and more likely to be helped by an early course of ECT. The American Psychiatric Association pointed in that direction when, in 2001, it urged that ECT be considered as the first rather than last treatment option for patients who are suicidal or suffer severe medical illness. It did not stop there. The elderly, physically debilitated, and pregnant women also may need ECT as a frontline therapy. So may people with severe depression together with psychosis, mania with psychosis, and catatonia. To do otherwise for those and others, says the APA, "may deprive patients of an effective treatment, may delay response and prolong suffering, and may possibly contribute to treatment resistance."

If it were up to Dr. Leon Rosenberg, who credits ECT with restoring his health if not saving his life, the procedure would be available to all patients and used sooner by more of them. "I wonder what would have happened to me if I hadn't been referred to one of the small number of hospitals that offers ECT," says the former dean of Yale Medical School. "The thing that is going to bring ECT back to where it belongs is simply the slow and steady accumulation of data and of anecdotes that support the idea that it is both safe and effective.

"I have little doubt that ECT will be used more widely in the future than it is now. It simply is too beneficial to be used as a last resort."

Nine

I FORGET

I still can't remember Paris. Oh, I have clear images of the city, its cathedrals, patisseries, and bright lights. It's one particular trip I can't remember. Michael and I stayed in a little pension. The concierge sent us to a different restaurant every night. It was magnificently romantic. That's what Michael says, and he rarely gets sentimental like that. I have to take his word. I don't recall a bit of it, not the hotel, the food, or even being there. The trip was a week before our thirty-eighth wedding anniversary, a week before my first ECT. The memory vanished, forever I presume, when they channeled electricity into my brain.

It is a price I was told I might have to pay. I did it willingly. I would do it again.

Memory loss is ECT's most feared side effect. It is what the public hears about most often, and what critics complain about most loudly. I believe anyone who says her or his ability to remember has been permanently damaged, and that big chunks of their lives were lost. Who would make up something like that?

On the other hand, most ECT patients I know have had milder memory problems, and some have had none. As for the situation I know best, mine, the memory issues are real but manageable.

Let me tell you what that loss is like. I forget telephone numbers, including ones I dial all the time like my son John's or my friend Anne Fetherman's. I sometimes don't know where I am supposed to go or at what time. Roger Weiss says that a couple times after I had ECT, I showed up to our therapy sessions confused or did not show at all. I don't remember that, either. Following my first few sets of ECT I couldn't remember how to get places I should have known, like from our house in Brookline to Northeastern University, where Michael teaches. I had driven it hundreds and hundreds of times. I would get into the car and think, "Where do I go?" I'd park on Huntington Avenue, not far from his office, call him, and have him direct me the rest of the way.

What embarrasses me most is forgetting people's names. I live in a political world. My remembering someone may be only mildly important to them but it is really important to me. It seems disrespectful for me not to, like that person didn't count enough to register. After ECT I still go to receptions, dinners, and other public events, with Michael or on my own, but I generally am not on my game. I can justify it by saying it is easy to forget some among the hundreds of people I meet, and that people would understand if they knew I had just gotten a serious medical procedure. I don't tell most people, although increasingly I do feel comfortable admitting that I simply do not remember their names. They assume it's age-related. Worse is that I sometimes forget commitments I make to help people. I tell a refugee from Cambodia that I will call the State Department on his behalf. I tell a friend of a friend that I know just the surgeon for her, or lawyer, or psychiatrist. Stepping in like that is my MO, it is how I try to make some small difference in their lives and my world. Then I don't make the call or get back to them with the name. Promising it, then not doing it because I don't remember, is terrible. They must think I'm a ditz, or maybe insincere.

Things I lose generally come back. I didn't remember anything about the movie *A Beautiful Mind* until a year after I saw it, when my son John rented the videotape. Likewise Michael often has to remind me about people we will be seeing socially, although as soon as I see them I generally remember who they are and how we met. Cues like that are critical for people like me whose recall is impaired but not destroyed. Other memories I prefer to lose, including those about the depression I was suffering. I'll ask Michael whether I really was bad enough to justify ECT. He'll tell me that if I had gone without it another week I would have ended up in bed, in the middle of the day, drunk. But there are some memories—of meetings I have attended, people's homes I have visited—that I don't want to lose but can't help it. They generally involve things I did two weeks before and two weeks after ECT. Often they are just wiped out.

Paris is one of those, and I really, really want it back. Michael used to tease me about not remembering, saying it was my way of ensuring a return trip. He and I did go back earlier this year, four years and a month after our first trip in 2001. I know the blackout from that first visit was total, but I fully expected that being back would jog my memory. It didn't. At the airport nothing looked familiar. While I had a glimmer of recollection at the park near the hotel, it never grew. I remembered nothing at the hotel. I didn't remember Notre Dame, the Left Bank, the Seine, Champs Elysees, the Picasso Museum, the D'Orsay, or the Arc de Triomphe. I don't remember our taking long walks to those places, which Michael says we did on our first trip. I know that if I had remembered our hotel, I never would have agreed to book it again. It had a tiny lobby and a tiny room with a tiny closet.

Cramped isn't my style. Everything else on the recent trip was great, the way it always is when you experience a place as wonderful as Paris for the first time.

Paris convinced me that people who have ECT need to be prepared for some memories not returning—and for not being able to choose which they will be. Doctors need to be as forthright as Charlie Welch was with me that short-term loss is likely and permanent loss is possible. The consent form I signed, which I am told differs from hospital to hospital, also was forthright. It warned that ECT patients "often have a disturbance of memory" and "may experience difficulty in learning new information." While memory problems "will most likely subside within several weeks," the statement reads, "a small minority of patients, perhaps 1 in 100, report problems in memory that persist for months or even years after the last treatment."

The good news for me is that the losses have been less noticeable, less severe, after my recent ECT sessions than they were after the early ones. Dr. Welch says he sees that with a lot of patients. "The brain," he explains, "in some way accommodates. Eventually it seems able to be more durable in the face of this ECT event." That sounds reasonable to me.

At the same time, I have learned ways to partly compensate for whatever loss I still experience. I call my sister Jinny, Michael, and my kids, asking what my niece Betsy's phone number is, what we did yesterday, and what we are planning to do tomorrow. It's not easy for them to answer the same mundane questions, over and over and over. I apologize prior to asking. I wonder when they are going to run out of patience with "Kitty being Kitty." I also keep a notebook in my pocketbook and write down promises I make. It fills pretty quickly. I live more than ever by my appointment calendar, consulting it so often the pages are frayed by the beginning of February.

When I was writing this book, working with my friend Larry Tye, he learned to send me e-mails spelling out in detail the questions he needed me to answer. He also learned to write and call to remind me, two or three times if that was what it took. I learned to jot down thoughts the moment they came to me. Together we went back through my medical records, which jogged some memories and at times seemed like I was reading about a stranger. Michael, my three children, my many friends, and my doctors helped us reconstruct other missing pieces of my struggles with drugs, alcohol, and depression. The stories in these pages are the stories of my life, but that did not make them any easier to dredge up. ECT, on the other hand, made remembering more difficult, but only marginally so.

Another way I used to compensate after ECT was not to drive the week after my first session. Now I find I can drive much sooner, generally within a day or two, although I never drive home from any of the actual treatments. That is a precaution anyone would take after a procedure requiring anesthesia. When I get back behind the wheel, instead of taking off right away for where I am going, I sit for a few minutes and think out just how I am supposed to get there. Where is that Pilates class? What is the best way to head to my son John's house in Los Angeles? Once I get on the road most things come back, from street names to turns I need to take. It's almost like magic, like a door that suddenly opens.

Just knowing what to expect helps me cope with ECT's aftereffects. I know I sometimes get a slight headache, so I have Tylenol ready. I know I will be sleepy at first but will have enough energy to do things later in the day. I know that I will want to go out to dinner that night, and so does Michael. I know I will need assistance remembering directions and other things. There's a predictability with this treatment that helps me to plan what my life will be like, and that makes getting ECT easier. That part I always remember and find reassuring.

The memory losses generally set in after my third session of ECT in each series. With my first ECTs, the ones that began on our wedding anniversary, memories didn't stay lost for long. The problems were more serious after my second set. It took longer for things to come back and I started losing patience. I presumed Charlie had been giving me bilateral ECT, the kind where they put electrodes on both sides of your head and it affects the part of your brain where most memories are stored. Charlie later explained that I never got bilateral. The problem may have stemmed from my getting seven sessions then, two more than during my first series. Since then there have been memory losses, but none really bad. Last year Charlie tried adjusting the current I was getting—using the form of wave they call ultra-brief. There was less memory loss but the treatment was less effective. Charlie is convinced we can preserve that memory benefit and restore our high success rate if he extends the duration of the stimulus. I am willing to try.

Sometimes I don't lose any memory at all after an individual ECT session or even a long series of seven. That is what happened when my old friend Sandy Bakalar took me in for treatment once when Michael was busy. She wanted me to relax afterward, to take a long nap before we left the hospital. I had to remind her that she was supposed to pick up her grandchildren and couldn't afford for me to sleep away the day. The other time she picked me up I was much more disoriented, enough so that she decided not to ask me for directions. That's the way it goes: variable and unpredictable. Hopefully someday soon the refinements they are making to the procedure will mean more of those good days for me and everyone else getting it.

It is difficult to know which of my memory losses are due

specifically to ECT and which are not. I know that all the vodka and wine I consumed probably made a mess of my brain and my memory. Being on amphetamines for a quarter of a century can't have helped. Doctors warned me that my addictions would likely mean lasting complications—one actually gave it a name: "diffuse neurological impairments"—long before I had my first ECT. They did not warn me about the long list of antidepressants I took, many of whose long-term effects we are just learning about and some of which are known to cause memory troubles.

Then there is the fact that I am sixty-nine. I like to forget that, but I know my age has something to do with my forgetting people's names, directions, things like that. Jinny goes through all that forgetful stuff, too, and she's fifteen months younger than I am. So do Michael and all my friends who are my age or older.

But I trust Charlie Welch's take on all this. He says depression like mine can make it difficult to concentrate enough to process things happening around you and store them as memories. Given the depth of my depression—along with my age, alcoholism, and history of drug addiction—he could easily absolve ECT of any responsibility for my forgetfulness. But he is too smart to do that, and too honest. "This is clearly an ECT side effect," Charlie says. "If these cognitive disturbances were due to depression, they typically would get worse and worse and worse as your depression gets worse. But your memory effects always are worst right after a course of ECT and gradually get better. We should presume it's ECT-related."

My kids presume that, too. Kara, my daughter, who is very upset by my loss of memory, says "at least some of it" has to be due to the ECT. John agrees that "some of it is age-related, and some is your scatterbrainedness. But some is very specifically re-lated to ECT. It's the way you ask about a thing that makes me realize that thing, that recollection, is completely out of your mind. It's not a dim memory, it's no memory. The loss involves pretty mundane things. You were supposed to be here at two o'-clock, but don't remember anything about it. You don't remember how to get here. It's a little disconcerting when you don't remember entire blocks of things that happened pretty recently. But these are minor annoyances considering that you are a much happier, healthier person."

That is my take, too. I hate losing memories, which means losing control over my past and my mind. It is a major side effect of ECT, but for me it's the only side effect, and it is less of a problem than it used to be. The control ECT gives me over my disabling depression is worth this relatively minor cost. It just is. It's a quid pro quo, like everything we do in life. It is also easier to accept the losses of memory since I was warned to expect them, and since most of the memories come back. As my counselor Corky says, the choice is simple: Would I rather be depressed or be forgetful?

Ten

COMPLICATIONS AND CONTROVERSIES

*L*ove it or hate it. That is the way things have been with ECT since the 1960s. There are two camps, at war. One labels the treatment the best in psychiatry and says it is vastly underused. The other brands it brain-damaging and insists it be banned. Both argue their positions with a righteousness and pertinacity reminiscent of third-rail issues like abortion and evolution. Both say it is their way or no way.

Now comes Anne Donahue and her middle way. The forty-nine-year-old Republican lawmaker from Vermont entered the world of ECT a decade ago, when she came home to Vermont for a breather from her endlessly stressful job overseeing programs for runaway kids in New York and Los Angeles. She started teaching, and playing a game during her commutes on the interstate: "I dared myself how long I could close my eyes before panicking and opening them. It was not a direct attempt at suicide, but I wanted to have a terrible car accident so I would be taken care of. People would realize how desperately I needed help or care."

She confided in a friend, who convinced her to go to the hospital. That led to a series of hospitalizations and medication trials to treat the depression she had been suffering since the mid-1980s. When they failed, her doctors convinced her to try ECT. She got thirty-three treatments in all in 1995 and 1996, although how many, when, which kind, and what if any warnings she got beforehand are memories she can only reconstruct by looking at medical records and journal entries.

Her ECT was a triumph and a miscarriage. The treatment was able "to break the stranglehold of a seemingly intractable and severe depression." It saved her mental health and her very life. But it sliced into the sense of who she was and the life she had lived starting a full six years before her ECT. Her loss, like that of most ECT patients, was gradational: Memories from the year before treatment have not come back at all, those from two to four years before are hit-and-miss, while by six years out only random memories are missing. Gone are recollections of public events like the heinous Oklahoma City bombings, along with treasured private ones like spending a day with Mother Teresa and hosting a weekend-long celebration of her fortieth birthday. Most troubling of all are all the memories she does not realize are missing. Donahue is philosophical about the trade-off, comparing herself to a "cancer victim who must choose the horrible side effects of chemotherapy over certain death to the disease." What she cannot accept is the way the warring ECT camps either dismiss everything good the treatment did for her or brand her memory gaps as the ranting of an outlier if not a faker.

Most ex-patients would stop there, trying to work through conflicting emotions and focus on their personal recoveries. Holding things in is not Donahue's way. The lawyer and longtime advocate wanted to get out word about what had happened to her, for better and worse. She wanted to know why there was not more research on severe memory loss like hers and more effort to prepare ECT patients beforehand so they could cope after. So she pressed hospitals and state regulators in Vermont to agree to one of America's strictest informed-consent requirements for ECT, parsing the language word by word. She filed a malpractice suit against the teaching hospital just across the border in

New Hampshire where she got her ECT, agreeing to a settlement under which it adopted Vermont's consent form and created a more candid video for prospective ECT patients. She ended up as a reviewer of the American Psychiatric Association's latest book on ECT, and in 2002 was elected to the Vermont House of Representatives.

In the process she has become a pariah. ECT critics cannot stomach the good things she says about the therapy, including that she would have it again. Boosters are at least as disdainful, with Dr. Richard Abrams alleging that her complaints of lost memories are "a personal conviction, and one that is, like many other personal convictions, unsupported by any objective evidence." It might be tempting to accept Abrams's brush-off except that Donahue has undergone repeated EEG tests, taken neuropsychological exams at leading medical centers, and compiled other evidence suggesting that her memory issues are related to both her underlying depression and her ECT treatment. "I agree with Anne's assessment that these EEG changes and her retrograde amnesia are likely permanent sequelae" of her ECT, wrote her neurologist, one of several doctors to say that her problems could be or are linked to her treatment. Even more convincing is testimony from generations of ECT patients who report memory deficits, most for smaller chunks of time and less long-lasting but some remarkably similar to Donahue's. There are enough of them, with complaints enough alike, that it is implausible that they are fantasizing or fabricating the losses. The Vermont legislator, it is clear, represents a substantial minority of ECT patients who applaud what the treatment did *for* them but bemoan what it did *to* them, most of all memory loss. Even those who cheerlead for ECT generally have some complications to report; just as many who are bitterly opposed acknowledge that ECT did some good for them or someone they know.

It is not just patients who are eager to find a middle ground in the ECT debate, but a growing number of psychiatrists. They know that ECT is one of their profession's most effective remedies, but they also know that too many patients suffer side effects. They are adjusting techniques in ways that demonstrably minimize those losses, in the process doing battle with fellow doctors who insist that the treatment is safe and that attempts to lessen its impact on memory will lessen its impact on disease.

Donahue is working with those patients and doctors to carve out a compromise in the ECT debate, one that reforms the treatment rather than sees the status quo as immutable or seeks to ban it. "I was being told from all the research that my experience of loss doesn't exist. Yet I know without question what happened to me," she explains. "I also was discovering this opposite view that said, 'This is a deliberate and knowing fraud on innocent psychiatric patients who are having their brains destroyed by the evil kingdom.' I am not the kind of person who can believe that, either. I don't believe in massive conspiracies.

"I really felt in the middle of all this. I felt totally torn and totally abandoned."

That ECT causes complications is beyond dispute, although their nature and rate have been shifting over the decades. In the beginning, 40 percent of patients reported serious side effects like fractured bones and cracked teeth, most of which disappeared with the introduction of anesthesia, muscle relaxants, and a continuous supply of oxygen. Weight gain and menstrual changes are also less frequent today. Yet patients still complain of complications ranging from searing headaches and elevated heart rates to nausea, jaw pain, skin burns, prolonged seizures, difficulty breathing, and a resetting of their biological clocks, making morning people out of night ones and vice versa. The rate of serious medical injuries today is about one in one thousand patients.

Death also remains a risk, though much less of one than before. The death rate in ECT's early days was one in one thousand; today it is about one in ten thousand. That risk, the National Institutes of Health says, is almost entirely from the use of anesthesia rather than from the ECT it-self. Electric shock is one of the safest procedures where general anes-thesia is required, with a death rate lower than for just about any other surgery. Still, the NIH cautions that "the risk of death from anesthesia, although very small, is present and should be considered when evaluat-ing the setting for performing ECT." And that small risk is present for each ECT treatment in what is typically a course of six to twelve, since each is on a different day and requires a separate dose of anesthesia.

A side effect of ECT that is far more frequent, and more difficult to measure, is the loss of memory. Researchers began documenting those losses in the earliest days of the treatment. Repeated convulsions cause "mental symptoms" in "practically every patient," Lothar Kalinowsky, a student and disciple of Cerletti's, reported in 1950. "The most constant symptom is impairment of memory."

Over the years doctors and patients have filled in the profile of that impairment. The most common, persistent, and hotly debated effect, called retrograde amnesia, involves the loss of memories starting around the time ECT is given and extending back months or even years. Rec-ollections most likely to disappear are recent ones, which is not surpris-ing; it is unexpected that memories about political upheaval, man-made disasters, and other world events are more vulnerable than those about personal matters like a family illness or vacation. ECT can also damage a patient's ability to learn new material and form new memories, which is called anterograde amnesia. A third type of memory loss, nonverbal, can leave a violinist or dancer utterly disabled, usually temporarily. The last area of possible impairment involves non-memory-related reasoning. It is the broadest rubric—everything from recognizing faces to solving prob-lems and thinking creatively—which makes it the most difficult to pin down and the scariest to contemplate.

When will those memories and skills come back? Doctors typically tell patients that most past memories will return within six weeks, while the ability to learn new material could be back as soon as ten days after treatment. A new study from Columbia University, the most comprehensive ever, suggests that those time frames are overly optimistic for more than 10 percent of people who get ECT. In 38 of 306 depressed patients, memory and other cognitive deficits lasted six months, which was the time limit of the study. The loss was worst for the elderly, women, and those with lower IQs.* The good news from this and other studies is that most patients do better on memory and reasoning tests after ECT than just before, since it lifts the depression that clouds their thinking. And some of the lost memories involve trauma, anxiety, guilt, and other reminders of their illness that most patients want to see gone.

For all the studies and speculation, a lot remains unknown about ECT and memory loss. While ECT is a convenient and logical target for blaming any loss suffered after treatment, some of it is clearly a result of the underlying depression or other mental illness. Aging also causes forgetting for ECT patients along with everyone, as do medications taken before or after shock treatment. For the elderly, ECT's very success in treating depression can uncloak hidden dementia. Major depression is also the commonest cause of reversible dementia, and a successful ECT treatment can lift the dementia along with the depression. While advanced age, preelectroshock difficulties in thinking and remembering, and confusion after waking up from early ECT sessions may predispose people to problems post-treatment, there is still no reliable way to predict whether a particular individual will come out of ECT with a worse memory. Most frustrating of all, while scientists can point with some certainty to the odds of dying from ECT, there are no good numbers on the odds of memory loss.

One way of determining those probabilities would be to ask large numbers of patients about any loss they suffered, and researchers have tried. A study in Britain, involving 166 patients who had finished ECT

---

*People with more schooling and raw intelligence presumably can better compensate for ECT-related damage to memory and thinking, the Columbia authors say.

a year or so before, found that "a striking 30 percent felt that their memory had been permanently affected, although the majority meant by this that they had permanent gaps in their memory around the time of treatment, not that their ability to learn new material was impaired." Another study analyzed a series of earlier reports compiled by doctors and patients and found that "at least one third of patients reported persistent memory loss." But other reviewers raise compelling doubts about such self-assessments. Surveys by doctors can encourage patients to downplay their problems, while those administered by critics often self-select critical patients. "It may be a simple fact," one report warns, "that people are generally poor judges of their memory functioning and that such evaluations are heavily influenced by mood."

What do the big mental health advocacy groups have to say about the costs and benefits of ECT? The Depression and Bipolar Support Alliance calls it "an excellent option for people who have not found symptom cessation through any other method and who are deeply depressed and/or suicidal." The National Mental Health Association recommends it "with extreme caution," and only when nothing else works. The National Alliance on Mental Illness does not back any particular treatments but does acknowledge that ECT works, and says nothing that works should be banned.

Asking doctors is equally problematic. Most say they see memory problems, but that bad ones are infrequent and patients are more concerned about ridding themselves of debilitating illness than the limited memories they have to sacrifice. But ECT doctors also confess that they do not have the resources or opportunity to follow most patients years after treatment to see whether lost memories have returned. And patients with the most crippling losses, as Dr. Charles Welch of Massachusetts General Hospital acknowledges, "tend not to stay in our practices. They ultimately drift off—still depressed, burdened by memory deficits—and find other clinicians to care for them. On a clinical service like ours, we ought to be keeping track of those individuals who are lost to follow-up, to find out what has gone wrong with their treatment and what can be done to improve their experience. Unfortunately, that is not common practice in any medical specialty I am aware of."

Physicians and pollsters may have trouble keeping track, but individual patients are compiling their own scorecards of what went right and wrong.

Christina Heath is at one end of the spectrum, with nothing bad to say about her four to six series of ECT treatments. "Everyone always asks about memory but I haven't had a problem," the sixty-four-year-old Utah woman says. "Sometimes I have a tiny little headache or something where my jaws meet, a little pain there. I take a couple Tylenol and it goes away." Donna Orrin of Michigan does have "a little bit of short-term memory loss" from the ECT she had in 1992, "but I don't really mind forgetting the most depressing periods of my life. Also with depression you have memory loss, so you can't point to ECT and say with certainty that that's what did it." Orrin does, however, clearly remember how she spent "every moment of every day thinking about killing myself. At one point I was on MAO inhibitors* and drank wine and ate cheese, which I heard could kill you. At another point I took a hundred aspirin because I knew from a social worker that that could kill you. If it weren't for ECT I am sure one of my methods of killing myself would have succeeded."

Jonathan Cott and Karren S. Jones are at the other extreme of ECT outcomes, close to Anne Donahue. Since getting thirty-six treatments starting in 1998, Cott finds his "explicit, short-term memory debilitated, my IQ quantifiably diminished . . . my abstract reasoning and learning facility (such as trying for an ungodly number of hours to figure out how to work a new phone-fax machine or how to accomplish

---

*An early class of antidepressants that, because of potential dietary and drug interactions, is seldom prescribed today.

simple computer tasks) seriously impaired." His ECT was so ruinous that Cott recently published an entire memoir describing his experience and arguing against the treatment. "Even as I type these pages," writes the New York–based author of sixteen works of nonfiction, "I often lose track of what I've just written. . . . Someone once said that memory is like the ocean because from memory flow all thoughts and words. I am truly at a loss for words." Jones lives halfway across the country in Missouri, but her experience with ECT is a mirror image of Cott's. She forgot the terminology and everything else that went with being an intensive-care nurse, so had to give up that career. She forgot the birth of her granddaughter, which happened shortly after she got out of the hospital. And she forgot confronting her mother with a long-kept family secret involving alleged abuse by a relative. "My mother left and I haven't seen her for fourteen years," says Jones. "The one time I talked to her she said I should apologize for what I said. I said, 'I don't know what I said. I can't apologize because I don't remember.' She said, 'That's a convenient excuse.'"

But Jones renders a different verdict from Cott on her treatment: "The ECT I think helped because I was able to say things that had been kept secret. I'm not as depressed about them, they're no longer locked up inside of me. I'm not glad I had the ECT but it's okay that I had it. I think if I got really depressed again and knew I was that depressed, I would give my permission to do it again."

William Styron's experience with memory loss, like that of most ECT patients, lies between those extremes. It was in 1985, as he was turning sixty, that depression first struck the author of *The Confessions of Nat Turner* and *Sophie's Choice*. Like Kitty Dukakis, Styron was an alcoholic, and, like her, his drinking had acted "as a shield against anxiety." When he stopped drinking, "the great ally which for so long had kept my demons at bay was no longer there to prevent those demons from beginning to swarm through the subconscious, and I was emotionally naked," he writes in *Darkness Visible: A Memoir of Madness*. "Doubtless depression had hovered near me for years, waiting to swoop down. Now I was in the first stage—premonitory, like a flicker of sheet lightning barely perceived—of depression's black tempest."

As the tempest grew, Styron considered ECT, but when it subsided he was able to avoid the frightening treatment, the same way Dukakis did early on. Nearly twenty years later the depression came back in a form so punishing he was nearly catatonic. This time he got electroconvulsive therapy and "it definitely did help," says Styron, now eighty. When the despair resurfaced a year later, he had another round of ECT, with less encouraging results. The treatment robbed him of some short-term memory and the ability to think in the narrative fashion that had earned him a Pulitzer and a long list of other prizes. "The second time," he says, "I took more than I should have taken and it turned against me. . . . It had served its purpose and I went overboard."

∞

ECT doctors call memory losses like these tragic yet rare.

ECT critics call them brain damage.

The belief that lost memories and other ECT-related impairment are the result of damage to the brain is what most unites and energizes ECT's diverse opponents, from Scientologists to ECT "survivors," doctors to laymen. It is there in large type on the cover of anti-ECT books like *Shock Treatment Is Not Good for Your Brain* and *Electroshock: Its Brain-Disabling Effects.* It is palpable in their arguments that refer to ECT as "closed-head electrical lobotomy," compare ECT patients to "punch drunk" boxers, and call the therapy "a brutal, dehumanizing, memory-destroying, intelligence-lowering, brain-damaging, brainwashing, life-threatening technique." It is at the center of their insistence that the only ethical response to ECT is an immediate ban. It is their mantra, and it is scary.

But is it true? The case *for* brain damage starts with studies, many dating back sixty years. One in 1942 looked at autopsies of two patients who died after ECT. The first, the authors said, "offers a clear demonstration of the fact that electrical convulsion treatment is followed at times by structural damage of the brain." The second postmortem proves "that damage to the brain may result from relatively few treatments and that such damage may persist for some time after the termination of treatments, five months in this case." In another study, seven years later, researchers gave eleven monkeys as many as one hundred shocks each, then examined their brains in a laboratory. Most changes in structure, the authors concluded, probably were reversible, but some "structural alterations, no matter how slight, may ultimately become permanent. These changes, though small, circumscribed, and scattered, might, if increased in number, eventually influence mental processes" and explain memory loss and other "organic" side effects experienced by humans who get electroshock. Kalinowsky, the ECT pioneer, also weighed in, writing that "it is undeniable that the frequency of organic syndromes is an unpleasant side effect of electric convulsive therapy." Such "organic interference," he added, "may also be the effective agent in shock therapy."

Those and other studies helped convince Dr. John Friedberg, a leading ECT critic, that "the damaging effects of ECT on the brain are thoroughly documented. All told, there have been 21 reports of neuropathology in humans. It is interesting that, despite the importance of a negative finding, there has not been a single detailed report of a normal human brain after shock."

Friedberg is right that there were studies pointing to neurological changes in the beginning, when electroshock was given without oxygen to protect the brain, more treatments were given at higher intensity, and damage was more likely and less of a concern to psychiatrists and patients desperate for an effective treatment. Even those early reports, however, generally suggested that the changes were reversible. One group of researchers, writing in 1985—eight years after Friedberg made his assertion about no reports of a "normal" brain—used precisely that word to describe a postmortem study of the brain of an eighty-nine-year-old woman who had received more than twelve hundred ECTs over twenty-six years. The "neuropathological examination was normal" and the shocks "produced no observable gross or histological sign of brain damage," wrote the authors from the University of Louisville School of Medicine. "To our knowledge, this study reports one of the highest ever documented number of ECT exposures, and no ill-effects were noted."

In 1984, Dr. Richard Weiner of Duke University undertook a review of the ECT literature similar to Friedberg's nearly a decade earlier. "For the typical individual receiving ECT," the electroshock practitioner, instructor, and researcher wrote, "no detectable correlates of irreversible brain damage appear to occur." Dr. C. Edward Coffey, now at Case Western Reserve University and formerly a colleague of Weiner's, used MRI scans to explore whether ECT causes brain damage. "The brains of depressed patients referred for ECT appear to exhibit evidence of structural abnormality," he found, but there is "no evidence that a course of ECT produces brain damage." Most recently and convincingly, researchers at Columbia University used high-dose ECT on four monkeys to see whether brain-damaging lesions would turn up like they had fifty years before. There were no lesions. Columbia scientists offer two explanations for the radically different results: Either today's ECT techniques do not produce damage that earlier, cruder shock therapy did, or, far from being the result of ECT, the earlier lesions were evidence of the brain breaking down on its own in the absence of formaldehyde and other contemporary methods for preserving it in the laboratory. Either way, the researchers say, their study makes clear that "routine use of convulsive therapy does not produce structural brain damage."

The U.S. Department of Health and Human Services, the American Psychiatric Association, Britain's Royal College of Psychiatrists, and most other government and professional groups, here and abroad, agree. They repeat the explosive question that patients put to them: "Is ECT messing up my brain?" And they answer with an emphatic "no."

What they do not say, at least publicly, is that the very issue of ECT and brain damage is a red herring. Critics take the presence of damage on faith, or on the basis of evidence half a century old and scientifically iffy, using it to enflame the debate. Supporters deny any damage, perhaps too flatly.

The fact is that scientists know too little about the brain to know for sure whether changes they detect are harmful, are permanent, or might even benefit people with mental illness. The same is true for the cerebral effects of everything from psychotropic drugs like Prozac to a couple of beers or martinis. We do know that alcohol, sedatives, antibiotics, and other commonly used drugs can cause amnesia without necessarily causing immediate and extensive structural damage to the brain. All the back and forth on brain damage masks a more serious problem on which there is hard evidence: that ECT sometimes results in serious and permanent cognitive deficits, whatever the cause. Arguing about whether that constitutes brain damage is a distraction to most ECT patients. They know that their brain is malfunctioning, which is why they first came to ECT; what most want to know now is whether the risk of memory loss will outweigh any benefit in subduing their depression. As for researchers, if a truce were declared in the battle over labels of damage, they might be more motivated to dig into what really is happening in the brains of ECT patients.

Another issue that divides pro- and anti-ECT forces is whether electric shock ever should be given without consent. "Forced" shock is less of a controversy than it used to be, because it happens so much less. In Illinois today, 91 percent of ECT patients consent to treatment. In California, it is 96 percent and in Texas 98 percent. David Oaks knows firsthand about being treated involuntarily, having been forced to take the antipsychotic drugs Haldol and Thorazine when his family and Harvard University checked him into a mental hospital during his undergraduate years at Harvard in the 1970s. Oaks, who now heads a coalition of mental health groups called Mind Freedom International, opposes ECT under any circumstances but he is especially determined to see that it never is given without a patient's approval. "We're not focusing on where a patient is comatose," he explains, "but where a U.S. citizen says 'no.'"

Dr. Benjamin Liptzin, chairman of psychiatry at Baystate Health System in Springfield, Massachusetts, agrees in theory, but says there are situations where he and his colleagues feel compelled to give ECT even when the patient balks. That requires a court order in Massachusetts and most other states, and Liptzin says that "nobody likes to do involuntary treatment, whether it is ECT or forced medication. It's much more gratifying to work with a willing patient, where you can present the pros and cons. But I saw what happened to a patient with a history of recurrent depressions who was losing weight and not eating. I said, 'You really need to come into the hospital and have ECT.' He said, 'I'll come in and eat, give me another chance.' His son called later to say he'd come to the house and found his father on the floor, dead. He had gotten dehydrated and weak and his heart stopped. It's situations like that that put us in this situation of asking for a court order."

A more frequent and fundamental question facing ECT physicians is whether the information they give potential patients adequately reflects the procedure's risks. To their credit, ECT doctors were among the first in medicine to use consent forms and make other efforts to inform patients, offering a model that today is standard with any surgery and probably should be with any psychotropic drug. But the warnings they gave often were incomplete, sometimes intentionally so. "We prefer to explain as little as possible to the uninformed patient," a leading shock doctor confessed in 1949, explaining that telling patients too much might add to their trauma or scare them away from a life-saving therapy. Noble sentiments, but unacceptable by today's standards and probably those back then. Yet even today at many leading medical centers there is too little candor about ECT's risks, either because doctors do not want patients to flinch at a helpful treatment or do not believe the risks are real or relevant. A 2005 verdict against Santa Barbara Cottage Hospital in California found that it had failed to provide patients with vital information that, among other things, "ECT could cause irreversible, permanent memory loss." That kind of admission is rare at any hospital, as Anne Donahue found out when she had her ECT at Dartmouth-Hitchcock Medical Center in New Hampshire. She says her consent form gave her little inkling of the memory problems she faced, and an informational video she saw dismissed reports of memory loss as "nonsense." The new consent form Donahue helped draft, which is now used across Vermont as well as at Dartmouth-Hitchcock, strikes a balance, explaining that most memory loss is short-term, but adding that "there are reports of some people who have memory loss that is much more serious, long lasting or permanent. In addition, some people report difficulties with thinking and problem solving." The new ECT film takes a similar tack, dismissing reports of brain damage but warning that there are "rare" instances of "permanent memory loss where the patient may never be able to recall certain blocks of time or information."

Even when the warnings are candid and complete, critics raise another vexing question: Can consent be truly informed when the person giving it is sick enough to need electroshock? Not according to a series of follow-up studies. In cases where patients and their families receive substantial information before treatment, and are glad they got ECT, they still say they know little if anything about the therapy. Authors of a French review on ECT in adolescents were surprised to find that "parents were unable to describe what the treatment involved, even though they found the explanations given prior to treatment to be satisfactory. . . . This point highlights how difficult it is to a obtain true and informed consent, when regarding severe psychiatric disorders." In a British study, just 12 percent of patients fully understood procedures involved in their ECT, 25 percent partially got it, and 63 percent had "no idea or only described the anaesthesia as the treatment."

Sister Barbara, the sixty-six-year-old nun whose ECT several years ago lifted her depression while robbing her of memories, admits that "I should have asked more questions. But I was in a serious bout of depression. I was doing everything I could to cope with the day, never mind to deal with this thing called ECT that I'd never heard of. I feel, looking back, like it was somebody's obligation to tell me about this procedure. I got nothing."

Barbara may in fact have gotten nothing, or, as she acknowledges, she may not remember what she was shown and told. In either case, more is needed than simply explaining to patients about ECT. Donahue suggests that doctors tape-record or videotape each patient's explanation-consent session, or at least bring in a family member or friend who can help the patient recall later. Warnings and the signing of a consent statement also need to be repeated during long treatment courses, and before and during long periods of follow-up ECT. Even more useful, as the Vermont concurrence form recommends, patients should be given written information before treatment on how they can get help afterward if they experience memory problems. And they should be encouraged to develop lists of things they may need to remember, as well as to ask a friend or relative to be their memory coach after ECT. "None of this was offered to me," Donahue says, "and it was the lack of information, as much as the actual effects, which made recovery so difficult."

If questions about brain damage and consent to treatment form the front line in the battle between ECT's boosters and detractors, both sides increasingly are resorting to rearguard actions that impugn the other's motives and underline its conflicts of interest.

A favorite target of critics is Dr. Richard Abrams. He is the author of one of the most widely read and optimistic ECT textbooks and scores of articles in respected journals. He was an adviser to the American Psychiatric Association as it prepared guidelines on ECT for doctors and others, and his writings were referenced more than fifteen times in the latest APA report. His writings are also referenced repeatedly on the Web site for Somatics, one of two U.S. manufacturers of ECT machines. What is seldom mentioned is that Abrams was cofounder of that ECT device maker and today is its president. The Somatics Web site does say it was "founded in 1983 by two internationally recognized ECT experts and Professors of Psychiatry." It does not name them. Some articles by Abrams disclose his tie to Somatics, others do not. The dust jacket of the 1988 edition of Abrams's text, *Electroconvulsive Therapy*, talks about his background but makes no reference to Somatics; the 2002 version indicates that he is "Director" of Somatics. A Somatics spokesman confirms that Abrams is the company's president but says he is "not at liberty to discuss" whether Abrams also is an owner. Abrams initially agreed to be interviewed for this book, then wrote in an e-mail, "I think I'll pass." Do his ties to Somatics matter? Absolutely, say ECT critics and even many supporters. Abrams himself acknowledges in his ECT book that financial motivations are revealing, although he is referring not to his own motives but to those of the anti-ECT Scientologists.

Abrams is not the only ECT doctor who has financial connections to the industry. Harold Sackeim, Max Fink, and Richard Weiner, three of the field's leading researchers, are among those who have collaborated with one or both ECT device makers—with any payments they received generally taking the form of equipment, speaking fees, or travel reimbursements given to them directly or to their universities. Few question the sincerity of that trio's belief, or of Abrams's, that ECT is a healing therapy. But Abrams's financial ties to the treatment are deeper than most, and he is one of electroshock's most unabashed advocates. Disclosing such potential or real biases is routine in medicine these days; it happened far less frequently twenty years ago, when the first edition of Abrams's textbook was published.

An equally apparent conflict is one involving the Church of Scientology. It spawned the world's best-funded, most effective anti-ECT network: the Citizens Commission on Human Rights. CCHR argues its case against shock in the media, in pamphlets and online forums, and in the courtroom. Yet it never mentions that Scientology, which gave it birth and continues to advise it, is financially competitive with ECT and other psychiatric treatments.* Scientology has developed what the *Wall Street Journal* refers to as "a lie-detector-like device called an E-meter, which is used to treat mental problems often at hundreds of dollars per session." Scientology and CCHR officials undoubtedly believe in E-meters the same way Abrams does in Somatics's ECT machines, but they, like him, have a responsibility to divulge monetary interests that could bias their judgment. Not only does it offer a competing treatment, Scientology bills its "modern science of mental health," which it calls Dianetics, as an antidote to ECT. Dianetics claims that its spiritual healing system can alleviate unwanted emotions, irrational fears, and psychosomatic illnesses. "In shock cases, such as electric shock," writes Scientology founder L. Ron Hubbard, "tissue may have been destroyed and the memory banks may in some way have been scrambled, the time track may be altered and other conditions may exist. In all such iatrogenic alterations, the results of Dianetics must be considered equivocal. **But in all such cases, particularly those of electric shock, Dianetics should be used in every possible way in an effort to improve the patient.**"

Whether because of conflict or conscience, compromise is unlikely between ECT doctors and equally true-believing critics. Their takes on electroshock, psychiatry, and the world in general are too divergent, their positions too entrenched, their commitment to their side too burning. Supporters say ECT is so valuable for so many desperately sick patients that it must be preserved and expanded even if it leaves some small percent with permanent memory loss. And they wonder how ex-

---

*CCHR says on its Web site that it is "proud to have been founded by the Church of Scientology" in 1969. While it now is "an independent organization," the site adds, "CCHR members work closely with Church members on social reform issues and consult with the Church's social reform or human rights departments." The Web pages also make clear that the Church and CCHR share a determined opposition to ECT and that CCHR "was formed to investigate and expose psychiatric violations of human rights and to clean up the field of mental healing."

patients who make a career of battling electroshock are able to remember every detail of their memory loss without remembering a single lost memory. Anti-ECT partisans say any drug with as many serious side effects as ECT would have been banned long ago. Such risks, they add, are why malpractice rates for ECT doctors can be 50 percent higher than for other psychiatrists.

The former ECT patients who make up the core of the anti-ECT movement also dislike being lumped in with CCHR and its Scientologist founders, even if CCHR has proven its clout in passing ECT restrictions. "The focus on Scientology is a way of avoiding the issues. It's a distraction," says Leonard Roy Frank, whose bad experience with ECT as a young adult led him to devote his life to battling the therapy and the psychiatric establishment that administers it. "The real concerns are that it hurts people, it damages them. That's the bottom line with electroshock." Is there a middle ground where critics would be content with reforming rather than replacing ECT? Unlikely, judging from the proliferation of Web sites like ect.org, which features a "Shock Doc Roster" and ECT "Hall of Shame," along with other efforts of critics to bring down the treatment. "There can be no compromise on this issue," Frank explains. "Electroshock is an absolute evil. It must be abandoned or abolished."

∞

ECT doctors are battling among themselves with almost as much intensity as they are waging war with the anti-ECT movement. Here, too, memory loss is the defining issue—how seriously to take it, and what, if anything, to do in response.

That debate has been simmering for seventy years, but it took on a revolutionary zeal in the early 1980s when Harold Sackeim entered the field. The New Jersey psychologist's previous research focused on inquiries like whether the left side of the face is more emotionally expressive than the right, and what that implies about the brain. Questions he asked about ECT also had to do with the brain and behavior, but were less theoretical and more combustible. The treatment, he said, was better than any in psychiatry, "taking patients who are the sickest and getting them the most well." But it also was too "toxic," giving patients "thirty to fifty times the dose they needed" and unnecessarily scarring their memories. The way to save and spread ECT, he argued, was not to deny that Achilles' heel of memory loss but to make the treatment more forgiving. Why not try limiting the loss by lowering the dose of electricity, changing the form of electric wave, and shifting where on the head electrodes were placed? He was not the first to raise those possibilities; research on each dates back half a century. What Sackeim did was bring to them the same rigorous clinical trials used to test drugs. He masterfully tapped the deep pockets, enormous brain power, and steady supply of patients available through his posts as head of biological psychiatry at the New York Psychiatric Institute and professor at Columbia University, in the process authoring or coauthoring a stream of breakthrough studies. He was enough of a visionary to substantially reshape the way cutting-edge medical centers administer electroconvulsive therapy, for the better. He also was and is provocative and prideful enough to alienate Dr. Max Fink and other kingpins in the field, who accuse him of spotlighting and exaggerating memory loss to the point where it aids and abets ECT's enemies.

Yet even his critics concede that Sackeim and his Columbia collaborators have set the terms of contemporary debate about ECT for its practitioners and patients, starting with the battle over electrode placement. ECT doctors have known for nearly sixty years that they could reduce confusion and memory loss if, rather than applying the two electrodes to either side of the head as was done with the standard bilateral approach, they put one on the side and the other at the back of the head on that same side. This is called unilateral ECT, and it can spare the

part of the brain that controls speech and memory by shifting the electrodes to the opposite side.* The problem was that while unilateral ECT
produced fewer lost memories, it also produced fewer benefits in rooting out depression, mania, and other symptoms. That is where the Columbia crew came in. They showed first that simply generating a seizure
is not sufficient, that the seizure will not be effective in treating mental
illness unless enough electricity is used. Then, in 2000, they published
results suggesting just how big that unilateral dose had to be—six times
the seizure threshold, which is the minimum electricity needed to produce a seizure—to work as well as bilateral. At that level, the researchers
concluded, unilateral is "equivalent in efficacy" to a robust form of bilateral ECT—"yet retains important advantages with respect to cognitive adverse effects."

Newer findings by the Columbia scientists more clearly define bilateral ECT's shortcomings. Patients given bilateral, for instance, take more
time to recall lists of words and have more trouble remembering recent
personal events like their last out-of-town trip. And lost memories may
not come back for six months or longer. While bilateral "represented the
gold standard with respect to ECT efficacy" for decades, the authors
write, "there appears to be little justification for the continued first-line
use of bilateral ECT in the treatment of major depression."

Some ECT doctors are not convinced. They say that because bilateral
works faster, it ought to be maintained as first choice for patients who
are suicidal, along with others who need immediate results. "A good
practitioner discusses it with their patient, asking, 'Are you most worried
about getting better as quickly as possible or about memory side ef-

---

*The speech center is in the left side of the brain for 95 percent of people, so unilateral
placement normally means putting the electrodes on the right side of the head. ECT critics rightfully point out that left unilateral ECT also can cause problems, only rather than
impairing verbal memory it is more likely to damage the visual memory on which artists,
musicians, and architects rely.

fects?'" says Dr. Charles Kellner, chairman of psychiatry at the New Jersey Medical School. "Nine out of ten times they say they are so depressed they don't care what you do. They tell me, 'you decide.'" Fink goes a step further, glibly noting that "it's not a question of when you use bilateral. That's easy. That's always." The priority he assigns to this faster-acting form of ECT is the flip side of the lack of credibility he gives to reports that it causes serious memory loss. By contrast, the American Psychiatric Association says it is time for "greater use of right unilateral ECT by practitioners." Dr. Richard Weiner, the Duke doctor who has trained so many others to use ECT, says he now starts all but his most at-risk and suicidal patients with unilateral, switching to bilateral only when unilateral does not work. As for Sackeim, he says "we are reaching the point where switching to bilateral should require consent by the patient."*

There is less ambiguity on the question of whether or not to use sine waves. The consensus is not. A sine wave is the kind of current that comes out of a wall socket and was the standard in the early years of ECT. The alternative, a brief pulse produced by ECT machines, uses about a third less energy to induce a seizure, generating fewer short-term memory problems and equally effective treatment. Comparisons like those, first made in the 1940s and confirmed in a series of recent studies, led the American Psychiatric Association to conclude that "the continued use of sine wave stimulation in ECT is not justified." There is less consensus about using an even narrower, lower-dose pulse, called ultra-brief. Research is ongoing, but the APA, Sackeim, and others say it looks like ultra-brief can be as effective as brief pulse with even fewer cognitive complications.

The third big technical issue dividing the profession is how to decide on the right dose of electricity for a given patient. Dose is key. If it is too

---

*Such consent is now required in Vermont.

low, there may be a seizure, but it will not be effective in treating depression or other ailments. If it is too high, there can be more memory loss than necessary. Knowing what dose is low or high for an individual is difficult, because it can vary fortyfold. There are three ways to decide. The first and least precise method is to use a fixed, relatively high dose, knowing that it probably will work and hoping that it does not produce too many side effects. The second is to adjust the level based on factors known to predict the need for more electricity like advanced age, male gender, and a history of ECT treatments. Most formulas, however, account for less than half the variability in seizure threshold, meaning the patient is likely to get a dose too low to be effective or substantially higher than she needs. The third approach, which the APA says is most certain, is to test various levels to find the lowest needed to induce a seizure. The doctor then multiplies that dose by a factor of six if using unilateral ECT, or two and a half with bilateral, to ensure a seizure strong enough to be successful. The downsides of this titration technique are that, while setting the threshold, the patient will have one seizure that is extra and unrelated to treatment, and she could have several shots of electricity that fail to generate a convulsion. The upside is that the patient is likely to get no more electricity than needed during the six to twelve treatments that follow.

The last debate on technique is over frequency. In Canada, Britain, and much of the rest of Europe, ECT is given twice a week. In the United States, Ireland, and India, it typically is done three times a week. The former is less likely to produce memory loss; the latter generates quicker relief from depression and other symptoms and shorter, cheaper stays for anyone getting ECT as an inpatient. The APA and most other psychiatric bodies say the choice should be based on whether someone is more interested in a speedy response than in avoiding possible complications. Those authorities also caution against more than three treatments a week.

Compelling studies and logic may influence the APA to recommend various ECT techniques, but not everyone pays attention. In a nation-wide survey published in 1993, only 39 percent of doctors used the titrating method of determining dose, 49 percent employed the formula approach that APA says "can be justified" but is not as precise, and 12 percent used the risky fixed-dose system. A comparable disconnect between what the experts recommend and what doctors do was found in a more recent study involving fifty-nine facilities administering ECT in the New York area. Eleven percent of those patients still were receiving high-energy sine wave stimulation, 75 percent got the more memory-impairing bilateral ECT, and barely half used titration to determine dose. "We're not doing a good enough job, for whatever reason, in educating the medical profession about modern ECT," says Dr. Sarah Lisanby, director of brain stimulation at Columbia and a key member of the team that helped develop those modern methods. "The breakthrough has already been made but people don't know it."

If the debate over ECT technique divides ECT doctors, imagine what it does to patients. Most are so preoccupied with the decision about having electroshock they are not even aware there is an issue about what form to choose. That is especially true for those on death's door, who "wonder why they are even having this discussion about cognitive side effects," says Dr. W. Vaughn McCall, president of the Association for Convulsive Therapy. "In that situation it's high dose bilateral and damn the torpedoes. I used to be apologetic for the side effects of ECT, afraid it might scare people off. What's fascinating to me is that it doesn't. These people are so miserable." Interviews with scores of patients confirm a desperation for anything that might make them better. "I would have taken a shot at a lobotomy, compared to the way I was living," recalled an ECT patient from Boston. Another from Los Angeles said he "would have amputated one of my limbs." Most sympathize with survivor-critics but not with their call to ban ECT. Most also say that as hard as it is to handle memory loss, staying sick is worse.

Still, even patients who cheerlead ECT are showing a more nuanced approach to it. The longer they get the treatment the more sophisticated they become about its incarnations—from bilateral to uni, brief pulse to ultra-brief. They can see how each affects them memory-wise. They also can see that the loss they took as the price of getting better need not be. Increasingly they are telling the doctor what they want rather than trusting his choice. Many who have read or heard of it are taken in by Sackeim's vision of a kinder, gentler generation of electroshock.

Susan Kadis had both kinds of ECT, bilateral and unilateral, the former in 1990 and the latter thirteen years later. While no fan of the treatment, she was so depressed that "I honestly believe I would have died if I hadn't had it." She also saw huge differences between unilateral, which left her with memory loss about personal matters but able to function at work, and bilateral, where "I couldn't remember how to use my computer, how to run programs, how to put paper in the printer." Kadis, who is fifty-one and works for the State of Maryland as a mental health consumer advocate, offers this advice for anyone considering ECT: "Unless there's a damn good reason, they should always start out with the least of two evils, unilateral. If you can get that, why go gangbusters with bilateral? There's going to be a series of ECTs and you can always change to bilateral if you need to. It's kind of like, why would you start out with morphine when maybe Tylenol will work?"

Steven A. Katz, a California-based engineer, is another test case for unilateral versus bi. Bilateral left him "zoned out and really having a hard time. It was intolerable." Unilateral was "much more pleasant. My only memory problems then were around the week or two prior to and after the ECT." When anyone asks about his experience with ECT, Katz says, "I say absolutely, 150 percent, do it . . . but I would definitely say do the unilateral."

Anne Donahue wants to build on experiences like Kadis's, Katz's, and her own. She knows the challenge of getting people sick enough to need ECT to absorb her advice, especially when it contradicts what their doctors are saying. She has worked with Sackeim enough to know the resistance he has encountered in taking such a high-profile role with ECT, including what he says are more than fifty death threats. Even so, Donahue is trying. She has written "A Basic Layperson's Guide to Decision-Making about ECT." She fields calls from people considering the treatment, in her role as a legislator in Vermont and as editor of *Counterpoint,* a journal on mental health. And she penned a long essay about her experiences for the *Journal of ECT,* challenging the profession to rejoice in ECT's amazing benefits, but to stop exaggerating its effectiveness or denying its memory effects.

The first advice she gives people contemplating the treatment is "go in with your eyes open. . . . ECT is a critically vital treatment for buying some time, but it's not a cure. If a doctor tells you that you are unlikely to have any memory loss, that it's not a big concern, then run out that door because that doctor is not up to date." There are ways to prepare for memory loss, she says, including getting an MRI done before treatment so you have a baseline against which to compare any effects on the brain afterward. Most important, patients have to know at least the basics about ECT before they agree to a particular treatment strategy. "If the doctor wants to start you on bilateral ECT," Donahue urges, "walk out that door. Also talk to them about dose titration, know if they are familiar with the latest research. The problem is that most doctors around the country still are on automatic pilot and are not utilizing any of that research."

Eleven

A SHOCK TO THE SYSTEM

I don't know how ECT works. I don't really care.

I know that sounds myopic, maybe even close-minded. But I think it's a feeling shared by most people who have sunk as deep as I had. We don't know how antidepressants work, or antipsychotics. We don't know whether Freud was right, or Jung, or any of the other fathers of psychology. What we know is that the brain is complicated, and that ours is out of sync. We are better than any psychiatrist at measuring whether a remedy works and what its side effects are. It's the *why* that eludes us but does not particularly bother us.

Michael is different. He is a problem solver and a lateral thinker. He likes clear-cut, measurable answers. That is one reason why he is skeptical of therapy. It's too squishy. It probably also is why he was open to ECT, despite the sour taste left by his brother Stelian's experience. He knew convulsive treatment is something concrete, with biological or chemical roots. He saw that when I drank myself into unconsciousness it shocked my whole system, body and mind, and even while it was poisoning me it oftentimes shook me out of despair. He put two and two together, wondering whether ECT works the same as alcohol, jolting me out of my blues. It's an unscientific explanation, but then the scientists have yet to figure just what mechanisms are involved. It makes sense and fulfills his need to know.

All I know is that ECT breaks me out of my depressive cycle. It makes me feel like I am taking concrete, constructive action, which in itself is positive. I feel in control, hopeful. I have been grasping for solutions, and this one is paying off. As long as I know the effect, I can live without knowing the cause. I never was very good at biology and was even worse with chemistry, so I can only follow distantly the theories about brain chemistry and what those neurons do when they are sparked by electricity. Michael might be right. It might be as simple as shocking me back into balance. I hate the word "shock" because it scares so many people away, conjuring up memories of ECT's darkest days and embellished images from movies like *One Flew Over the Cuckoo's Nest*. But shocking or jolting sure sounds like what is happening to me, whether or not it is scientifically accurate.

I know that critics insist ECT causes brain damage. I don't feel like my brain is damaged. I'm also not sure what damage means. I presume electroconvulsion is changing something in my head. If someone wants to label that damage, so be it. I prefer to trust Charlie and my other doctors, who say there's no evidence of long-term harm and compelling evidence that sending electricity into the brain does something to straighten out its circuitry. I feel naïve accepting anything on faith, but trust is essential for any of us getting treatments that medicine can't fully explain. And the critics can't take away the most essential fact: ECT works for me. It makes me better.

Speaking of detractors, they are part of the reason I wanted to write this book. They have strong opinions, and voice them everywhere. They are all over the Internet. They speak out on TV, in newspapers, in books. They have the right to voice their opinions and express their deep doubts about ECT, especially if they have had it and were hurt by it. The problem is that lots of people considering the procedure think that is the only voice out there. So does the public. Both presume, with good reason, that most ex-patients are critical because all they hear is the bad.

I know, because dozens of people have come to me looking for advice. Some had read in the *Boston Globe* or other papers about my getting ECT, and called or wrote to see if I could tell them how it works. Michael counsels many of his students at Northeastern and UCLA who have depression, and he sends some to me to discuss ECT. Most have a head full of secondhand horror stories, about memories obliterated and lives ruined. Most also are desperate for something that will relieve their despair. I don't offer a panacea. I do offer one person's positive experience with the treatment.

I have offered it to enough people informally and in public talks that I am convinced there is a need to get the word out more broadly. Journalists also keep calling me whenever they are reporting on ECT, enough so that I feel it is important to get my story printed in my own words. That is what I am trying to do here, to tell my story clearly and concisely, alongside a medical story and interviews with scores of other ECT patients.

Another reason I am doing this is because of the stigma attached to the illness and the treatment. The mentally ill have enough to worry about, and shouldn't decide on a therapy based on what other people will think. That isn't fair. I know about the stigma because I was caught up in it. For the first year or two that I was getting ECT I didn't tell anyone but my immediate family and closest friends, and I swore all of them to secrecy. I was sure people would think I had gone totally batty if they knew I was getting electric shock treatment. We need to erase those slurs and silence those whispers. People with mental illness have a right to know what is available and decide based on a full airing of views. They need to know that most psychiatrists think ECT can be a brilliant treatment for people who have run out of options. They need to know that many patients do too, including me.

It is not easy to go public this way. I know what I am in for because I have done it before, with my drug habit, then my drinking. This is harder. That's partly because it means retelling and reliving the horrible stories of pill popping and drinking, of railing at my son and having my husband find me lying in my vomit. Worse still is the subject of my new revelation. Society finally accepts that drug addiction is a disease. Same with alcoholism. More and more people with those afflictions are speaking out—about their sickness and their treatment—and being applauded for doing so. Not so with ECT. Bad enough that my illness is mental, but that my preferred remedy is electroshock simply is too much. ECT hasn't made it into the mainstream. It isn't considered "okay." It doesn't arouse sympathy, or consoling, but condemnation.

I fully expect to be attacked. I feel like I am putting a target on my back for ECT's many critics. And I wonder whether my family is ready for what this book will bring. Michael and the kids support me here, as always, but I know John, Andrea, and Kara have doubts about my taking this issue public. So do my friends. Sandy Bakalar worries about my "turning this bloody thing around and making it a cause célèbre." But she adds, "I know that's the kind of thing you do."

There's one more thing I do, or would like to. I want there to be support groups for people who are contemplating ECT, and for those who get it. I never heard ECT talked about, by counselors or patients, at Hazelden, Edgehill, or any of the other treatment centers I went to for more than a decade. Not once. I have been part of a support group for alcoholics that helped rescue me. The same happened with my drug problem. Why can't it happen with ECT, too? There are so many people with depression who are scared and hopeless and who meet to talk about their problem, but ECT seldom is part of that discussion. There is only so much they can learn from even the most well-meaning doctors, few of whom have had ECT themselves and some of whom have a tough time admitting and preparing patients for its downsides along with its up. We can begin to change that.

So let me be clear. I am saying that ECT worked for me, not that it will work for everybody. I am saying that we need to face up to ECT's risks and try to reduce them, but we also need to acknowledge its potential benefits. I am saying, more than anything, that talking about this is a good thing. There are too many people in desperate need of a workable treatment to limit any viable options. There is too much need for open discussion to continue the vitriol and finger-pointing that have characterized the last half century of debate about ECT.

Twelve

THE MYSTERY OF
HOW AND WHY

Think of it as slapping the side of a fuzzy television set until the picture comes clear. Jump-starting a car whose battery has petered out. Or calling in Roto-Rooter to unclog plugged-up plumbing. That is how patients say they think of their ECT, only what has clogged up, petered out, or is too fuzzy for clarity is their brain.

Imperfect images, for sure. But after seventy years of studying the brain and its response to electroconvulsive therapy, scores of the world's most learned psychiatrists have done only marginally better.

There are a number of compelling hypotheses on the wellspring of ECT's advantages. Shocking the brain to the point where it convulses paradoxically has an anticonvulsant effect, and researchers think that could dampen the flow of blood and electrical activity in a way that reduces depression. Or it may have to do with changing levels of serotonin or dopamine, mimicking the effects of antidepressant drugs. Some doctors see the brain as spongelike, with ECT squeezing it until it releases hormones, neurotransmitters, and other compounds that restore the mind's emotional equilibrium.

For now, these and other explanations remain in the realm of theory. Science's evolving understanding of biochemistry and genetics helps fill in the puzzle of how the brain works, but too many pieces are still missing to fully comprehend this most elaborate of organs. ECT patients are equally difficult to unravel or generalize about, with conditions ranging from depression to Parkinson's disease and treatment outcomes ranging from miraculous to memory-impairing. Experiments with rats, mice, and monkeys provide clues, but they are more useful for weighing safety than for calibrating mental illness and psychological health. More sensitive MRIs and CT scans offer a clearer lens into the brain that should help scientists pinpoint the chemical mechanisms and biological effects of ECT, but until then it remains a maddening matter of looking but not quite seeing.

"The black box still is pretty black," says Dr. Thomas Neylan, a biological psychiatrist at the VA Medical Center in San Francisco and former head of the ECT service at California Pacific Medical Center. "People are focused on different mechanisms of what's going on. They are looking at what's happening with neurons, with gene expressions, with dendritic nerve growth. But all that still is in its infancy as to why it works."

Does the mechanism matter? That depends on whom you ask. Scientists are eager to know exactly how ECT works so they can fine-tune it, and so they can answer critics who insist it is damaging the brain. Knowing what makes ECT effective also would help with a series of more targeted techniques researchers are testing to stimulate the brain without the need for full-fledged seizures and with far fewer side effects. Then there is the mystery itself, the conundrum that has befuddled psychiatrists since Ugo Cerletti's day of just why this seemingly barbaric process of shocking the brain somehow yields such healing results.

"Not knowing how ECT works," writes psychiatrist Keith Russell Ablow, "is hard for me to tolerate; as someone who has spent eleven years immersed in the study of science and medicine, I want to know precisely which gears of illness I interfere with. Strange that I worry little about the brain chemicals I set in motion with psychotherapy. I'm comfortable with intuition and insight. I'm a mind doctor. But when I use a machine and resort to electricity, I feel like a brain doctor. I wear my white coat. I drape a stethoscope around my neck."

Patients are different. To most, results matter more than the process that produces them. "We don't know why aspirin works or why lithium works," says Donna Orrin, a Michigan social worker whose eight ECT treatments lifted her out of depression and an obsession with killing herself. "I don't care why ECT works. I care that it does work."

$$\infty$$

Explanations for how ECT works have been offered up with conviction for seventy years, but they generally have been more enlightening about the scientific ideology of the era than about electroshock itself.

In the 1940s the therapy itself was cruder, with side effects that were more frequent and scarring. There also were fewer strident critics raising charges of brain damage, so acknowledging that ECT might produce damage along with benefits was less threatening to ECT's promoters. One of them, a Harvard-affiliated psychiatrist named Abraham Myerson, in 1943 suggested that "there have to be organic changes or organic disturbance in the physiology of the brain for the cure to take place" with electroshock. "I think it may be true that these people have for the time being at any rate more intelligence than they can handle and that the reduction in intelligence is an important factor in the curative process." Dr. Abram Bennett, who introduced curare to ECT, agreed that "mental confusion" was the key to the treatment's success. "This organic confusional state makes the patient forget his worries and breaks up self-consciousness and obsessive thinking," he wrote in 1949. "The reaction closely resembles that seen following lobotomy." Dr. Max Fink, ECT's biggest booster the last half century, in 1958 chose an equally unsettling analogy to describe how the therapy works. Repeated convulsions, he wrote, can be tracked using EEG tests and show up as "high-voltage, symmetric, slow-wave activity, occasionally with spike activity, which is similar to that observed in severe head trauma."*

Psychotherapy was the prevailing psychiatric model in those days, not long after Sigmund Freud's death and in the heyday of his influence. Doctors drew on psychoanalytic reasoning as another way to explain electroshock's effectiveness. Shock-related amnesia should be seen as "aiding the patients to forget their emotional problems temporarily and thus eventually breaking up the psychopathic pattern," Dr. Nolan D.C. Lewis of Columbia University told his colleagues at a 1942 meeting of the New York Academy of Medicine. "In the successful case the patient has gained a more complete control over the dominating psychopathological ideas, and the immediately favorable results are startling, even miraculous." Dr. Herman Selinski, a major in the Air Force Medical Corps, offered a slightly different psychodynamic explanation in a talk the following year at the New York Academy. "Shock treatment," he reasoned, "affects the psyche of the patient as a profound threat to his very existence. It reaches down to something primitive—we can call it the instinct for self-preservation—or ego instincts—or what you will—in the human organism." Rather than a negative development, Selinski saw it as leading to "early disappearance of suicidal impulses among the psych-pathological phenomena of the patient's mental disorder. One may speak of a reintegration of ego structure made possible by a violent shock to the personality."

So many were the early interpretations, and so bizarre, that one author

---

*It is precisely that sort of slow-wave change that has shown up in three EEGs she has had, spaced years apart, since getting ECT, says State Representative Anne Donahue of Vermont. The slow-wave activity was not visible in an EEG she had pre-ECT, Donahue adds, suggesting that it could be a marker for the cognitive losses she has suffered.

tried to pull them together in 1948 in a paper entitled "Fifty Shock Therapy Theories." His compendium explored twenty-seven biological theories to explain electroshock, along with insulin coma and Metrazol remedies. They might shake up the circulatory system, eliminate diseased nerve cells, or involve destruction similar to what happens with a prefrontal lobotomy. Another twenty-three explanations were psychologically based, arguing that the three therapies' effectiveness is a function of fear, amnesia, sexual excitement, punishment, or that "the patient sees in the physician a mother." The author, Major Hirsch L. Gordon of the U.S. Marine Hospital in Stapleton, New York, prophetically conceded that "many great drugs and curative methods began as (and some still are) empiricals and the shock therapies' usefulness would not diminish even if their mode of action were to remain forever obscure."

Maestro Cerletti wove in both threads laid out by Gordon, the psychological and physiological, in trying to make sense of the treatment he had given birth to a generation earlier. "It is extremely probable," Cerletti wrote in 1954, "that the convulsive attack represents a typical powerful reaction of terror and defense against definite stimuli that endanger the life of the individual. Considering the convulsive attack as a complex reaction preformed in the neuraxis with the obvious significance of a final defense of the organism against a given harmful situation, we believe that once such a reaction has been induced by whatever method available (we have seen why the electric stimulus appears to be the most suitable) one should allow the reaction to proceed normally in its entirety."

The most honest appraisal of the state of knowledge about ECT during its golden era came from California's Department of Mental Hygiene, which noted in its 1950–52 *Biennial Report* that "the exact mechanism by which electroshock therapy helps unscramble twisted emotions and thought processes is something no one understands completely even after years of continuing research. Nevertheless, the effectiveness of electroshock treatment is undisputed."

Our understanding of the brain has come a long way in recent decades, as have technologies for peering into that gray matter. A consensus has formed that ECT has little to do with Freudian notions of altering the ego or frightening patients back to health. Likewise, scientists now believe that while memory loss often accompanies ECT, the treatment works just as well without it and loss occurs whether or not there is healing. What is key is that ECT releases chemicals that make brain cells work better, although precisely how that happens is open to dueling theories.

The seizure is a centerpiece, although not necessarily in the way researchers thought. It might exert its helpful effect not through the convulsion per se, but by touching off an anticonvulsant response that reduces the excitability of brain tissue. "We all may have the brain structure and chemistry necessary to experience depression, but in some people, the brain does not release the proper chemicals to shut it down," writes Harold A. Sackeim, the Columbia researcher. ECT presumably does so by sparking a convulsion in response to which the brain releases an anticonvulsant substance—maybe a peptide, maybe a compound like serotonin that transmits impulses between nerves—that stifles the seizure and with it the depression. "The only reason we are producing a seizure," says Sackeim, "is to get the brain to stop the seizure. . . . An even smarter way to do it someday would be not to start the seizure at all and figure out another way to set off the inhibitory effect."

The hypothesis is compelling and harks back to Cerletti's quest in the 1940s for a shock that would produce results without producing a convulsion. But the puzzle remains as to the actual pathway in the brain by which the seizure—and ECT as a whole—works. "We know a lot about what ECT does through decades of research. It releases all kinds of neurotransmitters. It alters blood flow metabolism. It induces the growth of new neurons," says Dr. Sarah Lisanby, a colleague of Sackeim's at Columbia and chair of the American Psychiatric Association's Committee on ECT and Related Treatments. "Which of these is essential for the antidepressant response and which are irrelevant we don't know. We're working on that. We can see into the black box but there's a lot in that box that may not be essential."

Electricity is another key. Its dosage, waveform, and the density of the charge help determine how therapeutic it will be and how much memory will be lost. So does the precise place in the brain where it is delivered. Concentrating the seizure in the prefrontal cortex, site of higher thinking, is the best way to ensure that it is maximally effective, say Lisanby, Sackeim, and others. The best way to guard against cognitive damage is to keep that seizure from spreading to other parts of the brain, especially the temporal lobe that is the center of smell, hearing, and short-term memory.

Others see convulsions and electricity differently. Seizures work best in reducing depression not when they are controlled and set off a contained anticonvulsant effect but when they spread more diffusely through the brain, starting in the prefrontal area, then spreading through the cortex and subcortex. The more dispersion the better, according to this reasoning, which Dr. Richard Abrams, the ECT author and device maker, calls the "anatomico-ictal theory."

Fink is drawn to another part of the brain's black box, the hypothalamus, which releases hormones that mediate emotions. People with mental illness are missing certain hormones, creating chaos in their glandular system and emotional life. ECT, he postulates, sets off a cascade of hormones that somehow reset the brain's chemical and emotional balance. "Why does the patient get better?" he asks rhetorically. "She gets better exactly the same way you do when you go to a cafeteria. You've got a long list of foodstuffs. You pick up a ham sandwich, she picks up a cheese sandwich. A person who has melancholia has a deficiency. We're not sure which hormone she needs but we know that, like in a cafeteria, it's all there."

While those theorems differ in key respects, all share a sense that, rather than damaging the brain, ECT stimulates the growth of neurons and shuts down damaging mechanisms that bring on depression and other illnesses. Electroshock also appears to have more in common than previously imagined with antidepressants, especially the new class of selective serotonin reuptake inhibitors that make it easier for nerves in the brain to send and receive vital messages. In addition to mimicking those SSRIs, ECT may make the brain more responsive to the medications.

For all we now know about ECT, more remains unknown and perhaps unknowable. "Part of our problem in knowing more about how ECT works is that we don't know the cause of depression exactly," says Dr. Descartes Li, who teaches psychiatry and administers ECT at the University of California, San Francisco. "If we don't know the cause of the disorder, it's hard to know what the treatment is doing. We very much are functioning on an empirical basis here. We are shoehorning ECT into our theories on depression and the brain." Abrams is more philosophical about our state of knowledge on the treatment: "Modern neurohumoral theories of the action of ECT—even as formulated by sophisticated investigators with impeccable credentials—have not surpassed in conceptual elegance the 18th-century claim that things burned because they contained phlogiston; ECT awaits its Lavoisier."*

∽

Patients have fewer problems making sense of ECT. They know less about brain chemistry, and care less about it, which frees their instincts and imagination.

"The seizure just kind of dynamites the depression out of my brain somehow," one patient told *Time* magazine several years ago. Sherwin Nuland, a surgeon as well as ECT user, says it "was as though the electroshock had burned away a tightly coiled network intertwined in my

---

*Phlogiston is an imaginary element once thought to be released when objects burned. The French chemist Antoine-Laurent Lavoisier disproved the phlogiston theory by demonstrating the role of oxygen in combustion.

brain, constricting free will." For Andy Behrman, "after each treatment, my brain tension is almost gone and the pressure inside is reduced. It's as if a masseuse has worked the knots and kinks out of my brain . . . my brain has been reset like a windup toy."

That image of resetting emerges repeatedly, whether it is reconfiguring a clock, computer, television set, neurons, or the brain itself. Images like those matter both because they capture how patients feel about ECT and because they are as good as anything science has offered as a metaphor if not a mechanism for how ECT works. Rebooting is another theme ECT patients turn to, especially younger, more computer-savvy ones. Jump-starting works better for older ones, who remember the times they did that to spark life into an anemic car battery. The image that works best for Dr. Robert E. Peck and his patients is one where the need for treatment stems from being overwhelmed by a range of anxieties and pressures. What shock does, Peck writes, is "cut all the connections. . . . It is somewhat similar to a switchboard operator who, when overwhelmed by calls, can just pull out all the plugs and retreat to the ladies' room."

ECT critics offer up their own metaphors for a treatment they regard as rough, coarse, and cataclysmic. They see shock as the car battery that explodes when the driver crosses the wires during a jump-start. The computer whose hard drive erases when it crashes. Or the TV screen that comes clear when you whack it, but quickly fuzzes up again, with damage to the picture tube.

Dr. Charles Welch has heard all those allegories, the fawning as well as the furious, and feels none adequately captures the mystery and wonder of the treatment he administers to Kitty Dukakis and hundreds of other patients. "How we trick the brain to tune up the exquisitely precise and intricately complex ion channels, synaptic receptors, mitochondrial energy systems, etcetera, is of course the big story," he says. "It makes other kinds of tune-ups such as engines, pianos, or even computers appear moronically simple. It is exquisite fine-tuning of nature's most precise instrument."

Knowing how ECT works is not just a matter of curiosity. It is a matter of making it work better. That is what researchers are trying to do with a series of techniques aimed at stimulating the brain in a more focused and forgiving way.

The first and most time-proven is transcranial magnetic stimulation (TMS), which applies rapidly alternating magnetic fields to the scalp. To patients used to electroshock, TMS seems like ECT-lite. There is no pain or muscle strain, so no need for anesthesia, muscle relaxant, or extra oxygen. There is no seizure, and much less energy, so less risk of memory loss or other complications. A heart-shaped coil with copper wires attaches to the skull and delivers about the same current as a standard MRI test. All the patient feels is a slight tapping on the head, a sensation dulled by the bathing cap he has donned so the doctor can mark spots to focus the stimulus. All he hears is the thump-thump-thumping of magnets, like with an MRI, a noise dulled by earplugs inserted before the procedure begins.

What makes TMS different from ECT—and potentially better—is its efficiency. Magnetic fields are not impeded by skin, scalp, and skull the way ECT's electricity is, so it is easier to point the waves just where they are presumed to do the most good: the brain's prefrontal cortex. That is where depression seems to be centered, and where ECT seems most effective in rooting it out. TMS tries to replicate that effect, enhancing the activity of brain cells when they are inactive, calming them when they are hyperactive. It does that using a stimulus strong enough to induce a small electric current in the brain but too weak to produce an unwieldy seizure, which makes it easier to steer clear of the temporal lobe and other regions where it could be harmful. That elegant proficiency lets doctors administer as many as twenty rounds of stimulation at a time, five times a week, whereas ECT is so potent that it is limited to one shock per session and three sessions a week. And it means that TMS could be as therapeutic as ECT, but without the side effects.

Results so far comparing TMS to ECT are encouraging but not conclusive. Real TMS does work better than its sham or simulated version, although not by as wide a margin as hoped. TMS also has done decently in head-to-head comparisons with ECT. It clearly reduces depression, although apparently not by as much as ECT and not when the illness is especially severe, long lasting, or accompanied by psychosis. Thirty studies published over the last twenty years make clear that TMS produces little if any memory loss, as intended, and even some cognitive benefits. It has improved hand function in a limited review of patients with Parkinson's disease and may help with other symptoms. Still, there is too little data to say whether just stimulating neurons without a seizure can work over time, for enough patients, to give it a substantial role in treating depression and other mental ailments.

Dr. Alvaro Pascual-Leone is a believer. He has seen TMS work on four hundred depressed patients in his test program, along with hundreds more with conditions ranging from Parkinson's to strokes, and remains enchanted by its promise. "If you want to fill this glass of water," the neurologist says from his office at Boston's Beth Israel Deaconess Medical Center, "one way to do it is take out the roof above us and let the rain pour down. I can guarantee the glass will be filled, but it also will make a mess out of my office. That is what ECT does. But if I know exactly where the glass is," he adds, "I could get the water directly into it without damaging anything. That is TMS."

While most researchers say there are good reasons why the federal government has yet to approve TMS for anything but limited testing on humans, Pascual-Leone is more bullish: "TMS has proven that it works on enough people today that it is not an unreasonable and cowboyish approach. That doesn't mean a lot more research is not needed. It is needed. But it can help patients today."

Mike Henry is living proof. He begins talking as a technician hooks up the magnetic coil to his head, and continues chatting throughout his TMS session. Pascual-Leone runs a series of tests, looking for the lowest possible dose of magnetic energy that triggers a reaction in Henry—in this case, a twitching in the cheek or jaw that indicates the magnet is stimulating his brain's frontal region. The entire process takes ten minutes, the same as ECT, only here the patient is fully conscious, with no post-anesthesia disorientation, no convulsion, no hospitalization, no sweat.

Henry, a twenty-five-year-old senior at the University of Wisconsin in Oshkosh, has been flying in for treatment every nine or so weeks for the last six years. He had tried hospitalizations, a revolving door of them, to treat his chronic depression, occasional psychosis, and a series of suicide attempts that scarred his wrists and shoulders. He had tried "a barrage of different medications." He tried ECT, which kept him out of the hospital and alive, but did not provide lasting relief and sent him to bed after each session feeling groggy. He learned about TMS by accident when his mom saw a story on the TV news, and became the youngest patient ever in a trial of the treatment. "I don't have nearly the side effects I did with ECT, I don't have the grogginess," Henry says, explaining why he puts up with the forty-minute commuter flight to Detroit, a two-hour flight to Boston, and bunking with friends or in a hotel, all at his family's expense. He comes all the way to Boston because it is where he was accepted into one of the few experimental programs on TMS. If there is nowhere closer offering the treatment when he graduates, he will move to Boston, so convinced is he that TMS helps. "It has given me the freedom to continue my life and continue school. I have the flexibility of leading a life and not being so bogged down by hospitalizations and things like that."

Like most TMS patients, Henry says he would go back to ECT if he became suicidal again and needed a stronger therapy. Someday he might have another alternative. Researchers are exploring a form of brain stimulation that is more potent than TMS but weaker than ECT. It is called magnetic seizure therapy, or MST, and it uses the same magnets as TMS but at a high enough intensity to induce a seizure. MST benefits from the efficiency of magnetic fields the same way TMS does, letting it produce a seizure with a fraction of the energy ECT requires. Tests on primates and on fifty humans confirm that MST produces less disorientation after treatment than ECT, along with less amnesia and quicker recall of new memories. There was also a 50 percent improvement in depression, slightly higher than with TMS and slightly lower than ECT. But, as with TMS, the verdict is out on just how effective MST is, for which illnesses, and over how long a period. It does require anesthesia, and there are concerns about whether it can induce unintended seizures. MST also has not proven powerful enough to reach and generate a seizure in the all-important prefrontal cortex, although modifications of the device are under way that should make that possible.

TMS and MST offer hope that one size no longer has to fit all. The newer, more benign stimulation techniques sometime soon could be employed in a "staged approach—using the least invasive one that works," says Lisanby, who oversees Columbia University's brain stimulation programs. "We would start with TMS, then move to MST if that didn't work, then to ECT. The advantage is to save treatments with more serious side effects for people who need them." An even better system, she explains, would be to make the magnetic treatments so safe and effective that they could be used earlier in an illness than ECT, which typically is saved as a last resort. The ideal way to combine the three, she adds, "would be to find markers that predict who will respond to which. That is our holy grail. We aren't there, but genetic markers already are giving us clues."

Two other treatments—deep brain stimulation (DBS) and vagus nerve stimulation (VNS)—offer still more ways to direct catalysts to the precise part of the brain where they can help. But, unlike TMS, MST, and ECT, all of which are used sporadically, DBS and VNS offer ongoing therapy that could prevent relapse of depression and other conditions. With DBS, a pacemaker-like device inserted in the head gives off a continuous stimulus targeted at the frontal and subcortical regions of the brain thought to house the deepest-seated depressions. VNS also uses a pacemaker, but this time it is implanted in the upper chest and its wires are run to the neck, where it stimulates the vagus nerve that runs to the brain. DBS involves a substantially greater risk because of the precariousness of operating on the brain, but once the device is inserted it offers greater hope of working. VNS is the reverse: less risk during surgery and less prospect of reaching its target in the brain from its remote location in the chest.

For now, VNS is the only one of these new brain-stimulation techniques approved by the U.S. Food and Drug Administration, and it is limited to people with treatment-resistant depression. The others still are being tested. Only a few thousand patients have gotten TMS worldwide; for all the rest of the therapies, the count is in the hundreds. Yet even as the magnetic and pacemaker technologies are being fine-tuned, ECT itself is getting a makeover. One of the most promising approaches is called FEAST, for focal electrically administered seizure therapy. It is more powerful than TMS and MST, with greater pinpoint accuracy than ECT. The hoped-for result: a seizure powerful enough to help snuff out depression but not so strong that it spreads to parts of the brain critical to cognition. Researchers are testing FEAST on monkeys and hope to do the same soon in humans.

Studies also are under way to see if placing electrodes on either side of the forehead rather than on one or both sides of the head—a setup known as bifrontal ECT—produces the efficacy of bilateral placement without the memory loss that often accompanies it. A 1993 study on fifty-nine depressed patients found that bifrontal ranked between bilateral and right unilateral in treatment effectiveness but caused few enough side effects that it "should be considered as the first choice of electrode position in ECT." A separate study seven years later, on forty-eight patients, found that bifrontal worked every bit as well as bilateral in quickly treating depression, while those using bifrontal were spared the severe cognitive loss of bilateral.

Another way to reduce ECT's memory loss is with drugs. Animal studies suggest that as many as one hundred different compounds—from thyroid hormones to herbal remedies to mifepristone, the French abortion pill—can protect against memory effects. To know for sure whether they will work, however, takes more money than ECT doctors or device makers can afford. Drug companies, meanwhile, have little incentive to tap into a market they consider too small and potential competition to their pharmaceuticals-only approach to treating psychological disease.

Whether TMS, memory-enhancing drugs, FEAST, and the other new techniques will yield the kinder, gentler treatments that psychiatrists and patients have dreamed of for half a century is, like everything in this field, hotly debated. Do not count on it, cautions Fink, who feels the new technologies probably will not produce results in the real world anytime soon and are unnecessary, given how well ECT works. What really matters, he says, is keeping patients alive and pulling them out of their depressive or psychotic hole, not obsessing over memory loss that in most cases is limited and reversible.

Sackeim offers a different lens into the future. He sees the curious rise, fall, and rise again of ECT as providing critical links to the mystery of the human brain. The comparison he prefers is not among ECT, MST, and other forms of brain stimulation therapy, but between them and the pharmacotherapy that is the major alternative for most mentally ill patients. All the stimulation techniques—from the most shotgunlike, ECT, to the most refined, TMS—are substantially more precise and less risky than drugs, Sackeim argues, adding, "The problem with drugs is that you can't control where in the brain they go. It's a pretty lousy manipulation, which is why you get all those side effects. One reason why brain stimulation is so exciting is that you can stimulate different regions of the brain to turn on and off. It does it in a very targeted way."

Where does all this leave today's patients?

Ravaged as ever by depression and other debilitating demons, and expecting more as they see medical advances in other fields, they are desperate for a solution now. Hopeful as researchers are about electroshock's more forgiving sister treatments, these remain the subject of limited trials and continuing restrictions. Surprising as it is in today's quick-fix world, the only way to quiet the demons, for those who have no options left, is the cumbersome seizure-inducing therapy that Maestro Ugo Cerletti pioneered on the eve of World War II.

Electroshock is an imperfect remedy. But it is not the crude and sometimes brutal procedure it once was. It is faster and surer than drugs or talk therapy. It is safe enough to use on pregnant women and the elderly. It can wipe out memories, but chances are any loss will not last long, and even that may be preferable to the potentially deadly status quo. It may bring only short-term relief, but that can buy time for other treatments to take hold, and when it works, ECT can become an ongoing treatment.

It is ECT users themselves who will one day decide the fate of this treatment. As the shadows that have shrouded electric shock for more than three decades begin to lift, they are finding increased reason to hope. Contemplating ECT still makes many potential patients shudder, but the actual experience is turning more and more of them into evangelists.

EPILOGUE

T hinking about getting electroconvulsive therapy is unsettling enough. Knowing what to do next—whom to consult for advice, how to pick a doctor, which side effects to watch for—is at least as difficult. We explore those issues at length in this book, and we provide other places to look for information in the bibliography. We conclude here with more concise advice on the most vexing questions facing potential ECT patients and their families.

Can ECT help me?

It probably can if you suffer severe depression, mania, or the alternation between the two known as bipolar disorder. The more recent the depression and the more complicated, like when it is accompanied by psychosis or catatonia, the better the odds ECT will offer relief. It also may help with schizophrenia, epilepsy, Parkinson's disease, and neuroleptic malignant syndrome, although with those illnesses the evidence is less conclusive.

It probably will not work with obsessive-compulsive disorder, substance abuse, anxiety or adjustment disorders, and the less intense form of depression called dysthymia. Is your depression situational, stemming from an emotionally upsetting situation like a breakup or death in the family? ECT is probably not for you. By contrast, it does well with depression that is chemically or biologically based.

Certain medical conditions, from serious heart and lung diseases to brain tumors and lesions, raise the medical risk of ECT.

At what point in my illness should I explore ECT?

Doctors generally recommend ECT when antidepressants, antipsychotics, and other therapies have failed. They suggest it as a first-choice treatment for patients who are suicidal and cannot wait for medications and other slower-acting remedies, and for those who have used ECT successfully before. Electroshock is also prescribed early on with certain elderly sufferers, pregnant women, and others unable to tolerate drugs. A final group generally approved for first use: patients who are catatonic, malnourished, or facing depression that is utterly disabling.

The reason ECT is used as a last resort with other patients is that it requires going to a hospital or clinic and getting anesthesia, and it can produce side effects like memory loss. A reason many medical groups urge its earlier use is that it holds a greater promise of relief than any alternative treatment, and it generally works best in the early stages of illness.

How often will I need treatment?

A full series of ECT generally involves six to twelve separate treatments. Only one treatment is given a day, and doctors recommend two or at most three sessions a week. How many you get depends on how you respond to the early treatments. If you get better faster, you will have fewer, although most people get at least six. If you react poorly to early ones, you can discontinue the series. And if you are slow to improve, the doctor might suggest going to a full twelve sessions to see if that helps. As for whether you get treated two times a week versus three, think about the former if preserving memories matters most and the latter if quick relief is more important.

Once you are through that first series, you and your doctor should consult on whether to wait until symptoms recur before getting more ECT. The other option is to get ongoing treatments, tapered down to the rate of about once a month, to try to stave off a relapse.

It is important to be realistic about what ECT can do for you. It is not a cure, but it can offer life-saving relief. Depression generally is a chronic, lifelong condition, and if you stop ECT, symptoms may return the same way they would if you interrupted a course of drug therapy. You can treat them with medications, with ongoing ECT, or with a combination of the two, depending on what has helped you in the past and what kind of ongoing care you want.

How do I find the right doctor?

Ask your psychiatrist or internist. Ask your local hospital. Ask anyone you know who has had ECT. Ask support groups like the Depression and Bipolar Support Alliance and the National Alliance on Mental Illness. Ask Google or other Internet search engines (beware that most Web sites on the topic are strongly anti-ECT).

Finding a doctor who administers ECT is not easy in many parts of the United States. Finding one who has a long track record and offers the latest treatment techniques can be even harder. Then there are issues of instinct: yours, in deciding whether the doctor has the right blend of smarts and sensitivity, and the doctor's, in deciding whether you are someone ECT can help.

Academic medical centers, especially those doing electroshock research, oftentimes have higher success rates with ECT, but finding one near you, with a doctor who has time to treat you, can be a problem. The only alternative is to locate a community-based practitioner who meets the same high standards. Here are some questions to ask any doctor you are considering:

1. *Why are you recommending ECT?* Make sure the physician knows your precise illness, along with your history of other treatments, and can tell you how ECT has performed with patients like you.

2. *Do you offer unilateral as well as bilateral ECT? What technique do you use to set the dose of electricity? Do you offer ultra-brief pulse as well as brief?* (See Chapter 10 for descriptions of these techniques.) The more familiar the physician is with the range of options, the better. Even more essential is to find a doctor willing to discuss risks and benefits of each incarnation of this evolving treatment and to customize a program to your professional and personal needs.

3. *Can you tell me about memory loss and other possible side effects?* Beware of doctors who say there are no risks, because there are. Tell them what your fears are, and make sure they take those concerns seriously. Discuss treatment techniques that can minimize such risks, and what, if any, sacrifices you might be making in speed and efficacy.

4. *Where should I go for my ECT?* You probably can get it on an outpatient basis, providing you have someone to help at home, are not a risk to yourself or others, and have no medical problems that require hospitalization. Otherwise you would check into the hospital for treatment.

What will ECT cost?

A single session adds about $3,000 to a hospital stay and costs up to $2,000 as an outpatient procedure. A full series, involving six to twelve treatments, costs between $12,000 and $36,000. Those costs can vary widely, however, depending on your particular hospital and doctor, as well as whether insurance is contributing anything. Most insurance plans, including Medicare, do cover ECT procedures.

What about consent?

You should sign a form before your first treatment, and make clear that you want to be asked again for your consent if the doctor changes your form of treatment or recommends ongoing ECT.

Before signing anything, read any literature the doctor has on ECT and view his most up-to-date videos. Make a copy of the consent form. Have a sit-down with the physician to ask all your questions. Given the possibility that after ECT you will not remember any of that, bring a relative or friend with your for the question-and-answer session. Even better, bring a tape or video recorder. That way you can review the doctor's answers at home when you are more relaxed, and listen to or watch them again after you get ECT.

What other plans should I make before getting ECT?

Make sure you have someone to meet you at the hospital after your treatment and, if you are going home, to drive you. Also ensure that you have the next day or days off from work, so you can see how you react to the treatment and do not have to worry about functioning fully on the job.

Is there anything I can do to minimize memory loss?

Unilateral ECT, where the electrodes are placed on just one side of your head, reduces memory loss. Bilateral, the other often-used approach where electrodes go on both sides, may offer quicker results but with more memory impairment.

Some doctors are convinced that ultra-brief electrical pulses cause less memory loss than the standard brief pulse. Many are convinced that high-dose unilateral is as quick and effective as bilateral, without the memory issues. Number and frequency of treatments matter, too. The more you get, and the more often, the greater the likelihood of cognitive and memory loss.

Is there anything I can do to plan for memory loss?

Make lists of telephone numbers, security codes, and other essential information you might forget. Get the names of memory or communications specialists before beginning ECT, in case you want to consult them afterward. Tell relatives or friends that you might need their help. Make sure you will not have to make critical decisions in the immediate aftermath of your treatment.

Hopefully your recollection will actually improve as ECT lifts your depression or other illness. In the unlikely event you suffer memory loss that is long lasting or disruptive, precautions like these will help ensure that you have the support you need.

ACKNOWLEDGMENTS

Jill Kneerim brought us together, held our hands and edited our copy as we wrote a proposal, flew with us to New York to meet with publishers, and consulted endlessly and wisely as we constructed this book. She would have earned her fee with any one of those. With all of them she made clear, again, that she is our friend as well as our agent.

Michael Dukakis did what a sensitive spouse is supposed to. For Kitty, he offered support and counsel, as always. For Larry, he made the case that this was a book that should be written, and that Larry should be the writer. Lisa Frusztajer gave Larry insight, empathy, and more patience than any husband has a right to expect, especially in the first year of a marriage.

Several people took the time and care, under our tight deadline, to read and offer feedback on our manuscript. Anne Donahue, a savvy mental health advocate and state representative from Vermont, is also a gifted editor, as she showed in her comments on this book. Two other experts who provided guidance from the beginning, and valued critiques through the very end, are Dr. Sarah Lisanby, who runs Columbia University's brain stimulation programs, and Dr. Charles Welch, head of the ECT program at Massachusetts General Hospital and Kitty's doctor.

A trio of journalist friends—Claudia Kalb, Dick Lehr, and Don MacGillis—offered equally critical advice on our writing, reporting, and rewriting. So did media law savant Joe Steinfield.

ECT practitioners from around the globe helped us tell this story, and we are grateful. Special thanks to the ones we harassed most: Dr. Steve Dinwiddie of the University of Chicago; Dr. Max Fink of the State University of New York, Stony Brook; Dr. Charles Kellner of the Medical University of South Carolina; Dr. Harold Sackeim of Columbia University; Dr. Richard Weiner of Duke University; Dr. Tony Weiner of Lawrence Memorial Hospital outside Boston; and Dr. Beth Childs, commissioner of mental health in Massachusetts. ECT critics were equally helpful, despite their conviction they would not like the outcome. Thanks especially to Linda Andre, Ted Chabasinski, and Leonard Roy Frank, who shared their stories and their concerns. We drew here on the works of all the authors listed in our bibliography, but want to single out Robert Whitaker, author of *Mad in America,* who offered us his files as well as his feedback, and Dr. Matthew Rudorfer of the National Institutes of Mental Health, who helped us distinguish fact from fiction.

What to say about Megan Newman and Lucia Watson, our publisher and editor? Megan had enough faith in our project to buy the book and agree to personally oversee it. Lucia responded quickly and enthusiastically to our manuscript with ways to fine-tune the tone, clarify prose, and generally make it better. The tune-up continued, on everything from grammar to word choices, with Jane Herman's skillful copyediting.

Anyone involved in the world of mental illness knows that overcoming it takes a family, along with amazing friends. For Kitty, my children—John, Kara, and Andrea—answered my questions and Larry's about my illness and treatments. Then they answered them again. So did my sister, Jinny, and my brother-in-law, Al Peters. Thanks, too, to my dear friends Sandy Bakalar, Corky Balzac, Paul Costello, Anne Featherman, Dr. Wilma Greenfield, and Maureen McGlame.

From Larry's side, thanks to Alec and Marina for teaching me all that kids can about the things that matter most in book writing: listening, storytelling, and ice-cream breaks. Thanks also to my friends and enablers, some family and others who act like it: Dorothy Tye, Olga and Bill Frusztajer, Suzanne and Norman Goldberg, Donald and Ariela Tye, Mischa Frusztajer, Nina and Andre

Marquis, Alison Arnett, Andy Savitz, Marianne Sutton, and Philip Warburg. My appreciation to Marylou Sudders, who taught me more than anyone about the mental health system, and to Sally Jacobs, who continues to tutor me in writing leads and endings.

The Blue Cross Blue Shield of Massachusetts Foundation, primary sponsor of the medical journalism fellowship program that Larry runs, gave him the time he needed for book writing and, on this medical book, invaluable advice. Fellows from the program were incredible, too, as they heard from Kitty and Michael and asked incisive questions of them and Larry.

We hired a series of student-researchers over the last year. The ones who stayed longest and helped most were Juliana Seminerio and Mark Slomiak.

Last, we want to acknowledge the scores of individuals we interviewed whose depression, schizophrenia, bipolar disorder, and other mental illnesses were serious enough for them to get electroconvulsive therapy. You opened the most painful parts of your lives to us, total strangers. We are grateful.

NOTES

Preface

x **"a manic high like I'd never"** . . . **"At the time I said I would never":** Author interviews with Carrie DeLoach and Christine Elvidge, 2005.

Chapter 2. It's Back

9–10 **Collins-Layton could not wait** . . . **"Was I afraid":** Author interview with Barbara Collins-Layton, 2005.

10–11 **"I'm sitting in the waiting area":** Author interview with and e-mails from Sister Barbara, 2004 and 2005.

13 **"A procedure like that"** . . . **"with muscle relaxants":** Author interviews with Rhoda Falk and Laurel Zangerl, 2005.

14 **Women get more ECT:** National Institute of Mental Health, "The Numbers Count," March 21, 2004; Matthew V. Rudorfer, Michael E. Henry, and Harold A. Sackeim, "Electroconvulsive Therapy," in *Psychiatry*, 2nd ed., ed. Allan Tasman, Jerald Kay, and Jeffrey A. Lieberman (Hoboken, N.J.: John Wiley & Sons, 2003), 1868; Debra A. Wood and Philip M. Burgess, "Epidemiological Analysis of Electroconvulsive Therapy in Victoria, Australia," *Australian and New Zealand Journal of Psychiatry* 37 (2003): 307–311.

14–15 **Advanced age as a factor:** James W. Thompson, Richard D. Weiner, and

C. Patrick Myers, "Use of ECT in the United States in 1975, 1980, and 1986," *American Journal of Psychiatry* 151 (1994): 1657–1661; Joan Prudic, Mark Olfson, and Harold A. Sackeim, "Electro-Convulsive Therapy Practices in the Community," *Psychological Medicine* 31, no. 5 (2001): 929–934; National Institutes of Health Consensus Development Panel on Depression in Late Life, "Diagnosis and Treatment of Depression in Late Life," *Journal of the American Medical Association* 268, no. 8 (1992): 1018–1024.

15 **white, rich, and a Yankee:** "Use of ECT for the Inpatient Treatment of Recurrent Major Depression," *American Journal of Psychiatry* 155 (1998): 22–29; Richard C. Hermann et al., "Variation in ECT Use in the United States," *American Journal of Psychiatry* 152, no. 6 (1995): 869–875.

15 **poor are denied ECT:** Hermann et al., "Variation in ECT Use," 869–875; W. Vaughn McCall, "Physical Treatments in Psychiatry: Current and Historical Use in the Southern United States," *Southern Medical Journal* 82, no. 3 (1989): 345–351.

15 **"The reason":** Author interview with Dr. Jonathan Brodie, 2005.

16 **"It gets to the point":** Author interview with Marc Pierre, 2005.

16–17 **"my only recall":** Author interview with Geraldine Knaack, 2005.

18 **"Katie had lost":** Author interview with Catherine Steinhoff, 2005.

18 **"I just didn't want":** Author interview with Katie Steinhoff, 2005.

19 **"It is my personal prediction":** Robert L. Palmer, ed., *Electroconvulsive Therapy: An Appraisal* (New York: Oxford University Press, 1981), 2.

19 **A pair of researchers:** James W. Thompson and Jack D. Blaine, "Use of ECT in the United States in 1975 and 1980," *American Journal of Psychiatry* 144 (1987): 557–562.

19–20 **What . . . other prophets of doom could not foresee:** "The Royal College of Psychiatrists' Memorandum on the Use of Electroconvulsive Therapy," *British Journal of Psychiatry* 131 (1977): 261–272; "Electroconvulsive Therapy: National Institutes of Health Consensus Development Conference Statement" (1985): 1–23.

20 **reports suggested a robust recovery:** Thompson, Weiner, and Myers, "Use of ECT," 1657–1661; Hermann et al., "Variation in ECT Use," 869–875; Max Fink, "Is ECT Usage Decreasing?" *Convulsive Therapy* 3, no. 3 (1987): 171–173; Margo L. Rosenbach, Richard C. Hermann, and Robert A. Dorwart, "Use of Electroconvulsive Therapy in the Medicare Population Between 1987 and 1992," *Psychiatric Services* 48, no. 12 (1997): 1537–1542.

20 **"I was not responding":** Author interview with Julaine Siegel, 2005.

20 **the trend within the state [California]:** California Department of Mental Health, "Annual Report on Electroconvulsive Therapy in California," 1977–2002.

21 **The pattern in Texas . . . In Vermont:** Texas Department of Mental Health and Mental Retardation, "Annual Report on Electroconvulsive Therapy in Texas," Fiscal Years 1994–2004; Vermont Department of Health, Division of Mental Health, "Annual Report on Electroconvulsive Therapy in Vermont," Fiscal Years 2001–2004.

22 **number of Americans getting ECT:** Allen R. Grahn, "Summary of Presentation to FDA Neurology Panel, Study of Electroconvulsive Therapy Device Safety and Efficacy," Utah Biomedical Test Laboratory, October 15, 1976; Hermann et al., "Variation in ECT Use," 869–875; Prudic, Olfson, and Sackeim, "Electro-Convulsive Therapy Practices," 929–934. There are no recent authoritative studies of ECT usage the way there are with knee replacements or cardiac bypass operations. The figure of 100,000 is based on more limited surveys—of psychiatrists, Medicare and Medicaid recipients, privately insured patients, and others—along with author interviews of federal and state health authorities, insurance executives, hospital officials, university researchers, health care consultants, and ECT doctors.

22 **In England:** Joanne Greenhalgh et al., "Clinical and Cost-Effectiveness of Electroconvulsive Therapy for Depressive Illness, Schizophrenia, Catatonia and Mania: Systematic Reviews and Economic Modeling Studies," *Health Technology Assessment* 9, no. 9 (2005).

22 **In Scandinavia . . . "Very hostile anti-ECT sentiments have not been":** Author interview with Dr. Tom G. Bolwig, 2005.

23 **in the Third World:** Jude U. Ohaeri et al., "Tissue Injury-Inducing Potential of Unmodified ECT: Serial Measurement of Acute Phase Reactants," *Convulsive Therapy* 8, no. 4 (1992): 253–257; A. O. Odejide, J. U. Ohaeri, and B. A. Ikuesan, "Electroconvulsive Therapy in Nigeria," *Convulsive Therapy* 3, no. 1 (1987).

23–24 **The situation in Asia:** Worrawat Chanpattana et al., "Survey of the Practice of Electroconvulsive Therapy in Teaching Hospitals in India," *Journal of ECT* 21, no. 2 (2005): 100–104; Worrawat Chanpattana et al., "ECT Practice in Japan," *Journal of ECT* 21, no. 1 (2005): 58; "Abuse of Electroshock Found in Turkish Mental Hospitals," *New York Times*, September 29, 2005, 3; John D. Little, "ECT in the Asia Pacific Region: What Do We Know?," *Journal of ECT* 19, no. 2 (2003): 93–97.

24 **Adding up the numbers of patients . . . internationally:** Author e-mail from Dr. Harold Sackeim, 2005; author e-mail from Dr. Barry Alan Kramer, 2005.

24–25 **turnaround has happened sub rosa:** Vince Bielski, "Electroshock's Quiet Comeback," *San Francisco Bay Guardian*, April 18, 1990, p.17; Daniel Goleman, "The Quiet Comeback of Electroshock Therapy," *New York Times*, August 2, 1990, p.17.

25–26 **double stigma:** Joyce Jackson, "Electroconvulsive Therapy: Problems and Prejudices," *Convulsive Therapy* 11, no. 3 (1995): 180; author interviews with Marie DeRose and Rosemary Goodwin, 2005.

26 **"For months, in my conversations":** Martha Manning, *Undercurrents: A Life Beneath the Surface* (New York: HarperCollins, 1994), 165; author interview with Manning, 2004.

26–27 **celebrities who have gone public:** Veronica Burns, "Goodbye, Darkness: A TV Host's Odyssey from Terrifying Depression to Renewed Peace of Mind," *People,* August 3, 1992; Patty Duke and Gloria Hochman, *A Brilliant Madness: Living with Manic-Depressive Illness* (New York: Bantam Books, 1992); Lisa W. Foderaro, "With Reforms in Treatment, Shock Therapy Loses Shock," *New York Times,* July 19, 1993; author interview with Dr. Leon Rosenberg, 2005.

28 **"The attitude toward ECT":** Zigmond M. Lebensohn, "The History of Electroconvulsive Therapy in the United States and Its Place in American Psychiatry: A Personal Memoir," *Comprehensive Psychiatry* 40, no. 3 (1999): 174.

28 **"They say, 'There you go again' ":** Author interview with Dr. Beth Childs, 2005.

28 **Gaps in training:** Donald G. Langsley and Joel Yager, "The Definition of a Psychiatrist: Eight Years Later," *American Journal of Psychiatry* 145, no. 4 (1988): 469–475; Richard C. Hermann et al., "Characteristics of Psychiatrists Who Perform ECT," *American Journal of Psychiatry* 155, no. 7 (1998): 889–894.

29 **"Most residents get":** Author interview with Dr. Richard Weiner, 2005.

29 **survey of students:** Jeffrey L. Clothier, Thomas Freeman, and Lisa Snow, "Medical Student Attitudes and Knowledge About ECT," *Journal of ECT* 17, no. 2 (2001): 99–101.

29–30 **More gaps in training and retraining:** Richard C. Hermann et al., "Diagnoses of Patients Treated with ECT: A Comparison of Evidence-Based Standards with Reported Use," *Psychiatric Services* 50, no. 8 (1999): 1059–1065.

30 **"We had to retrain":** Author interview with Dr. Beth Childs.

30–31 **out of reach:** W. Vaughn McCall, "Physical Treatments in Psychiatry: Current and Historical Use in the Southern United States," *Southern Medical Journal* 82, no. 3 (1989): 345–351; Hermann et al., "Variation in ECT Use," 869–875.

31 **too often is used clumsily:** Prudic, Olfson, and Sackeim, "Electro-Convulsive Therapy Practices," 929–934; Joan Prudic et al., "Effectiveness of Electroconvulsive Therapy in Community Settings," *Biological Psychiatry* 55, no. 2 (2004): 301–312.

31 **"There are things where doctors":** Author interview with Dr. Richard Hermann, 2005.

32 **too little and too unevenly:** Tom Glen and Allan I.F. Scott, "Variation in Rates of Electroconvulsive Therapy Use Among Consultant Teams in Edinburgh

(1993–1996)," *Journal of Affective Disorders* 58, no. 1 (2000): 75–78 ; L.S. Stromgren, "Electroconvulsive Therapy in the Nordic Countries, 1977–1987," *Acta Psychiatrica Scandinavica* 84, no. 5 (1991): 428–434; H. Lauter and H. Sauer, "Electroconvulsive Therapy: A German Perspective," *Convulsive Therapy* 3, no. 3 (1987): 204–209; John Pippard, "Audit of Electroconvulsive Treatment in Two National Health Service Regions," *British Journal of Psychiatry* 160 (1992): 621–637.

32 **"If ECT is ever legislated against":** "ECT in Britain: A Shameful State of Affairs," Editorial, *The Lancet* (November 28, 1981): 1208.

Chapter 4. Serendipity and Science

50 **"Someone got nervous":** Ugo Cerletti, "Old and New Information About Electroshock," *American Journal of Psychiatry* 107 (1950): 90.

50–51 **"stopped breathing":** Ferdinando Accornero, "An Eyewitness Account of the Discovery of Electroshock," *Convulsive Therapy* 4, no. 1 (1988): 47. Time plays tricks even with scientists' memories, as reflected in the different accounts Cerletti and Accornero offer on everything from whether S.E.'s first jolt of electricity lasted one-tenth of a second or one and a half seconds, to whether he got two or three jolts that first day, to whether he eventually got nine or eleven sessions of shock. On all the important points, however, they were in sync.

51 **"The patient sat up":** Cerletti, "Old and New Information," 91.

52 **"An electric shock, shot directly":** Marjorie Van de Water, "Electric Shock, a New Treatment," *Science News Letter* (July 20, 1940): 42–44.

52–53 **"A patient hospitalized" . . . "if the doctor didn't":** Edward Shorter, "The History of ECT: Some Unsolved Mysteries," *Psychiatric Times* 21, no. 2 (2004).

53 **The ancient Greeks . . . The early Romans:** Stephanie Pain, "Lady Emma's Shocking Past," *New Scientist,* May 10, 2003; Cerletti, "Old and New Information," 87–94.

54 **Duchenne insisted . . . Sears, Roebuck catalog:** Ernest Harms, "The Origin and Early History of Electrotherapy and Electroshock," *American Journal of Psychiatry* 111, no. 12 (1955): 933–934; http://www.burtonreport.com/INDEX.htm; http://www.guthrietheater.org/pdf/sexhabits.pdf.

54 **Celsus the Platonist . . . Hungarian manuscript documented:** R. M. Mowbray, "Historical Aspects of Electric Convulsant Therapy," *Scottish Medical Journal* 4 (1959): 373–378; Alison Linington and Brian Harris, "Fifty Years of Electroconvulsive Therapy," *British Medical Journal* 297 (November 26, 1988): 1354–1355; Richard Abrams, *Electroconvulsive Therapy,* 4th ed. (New York: Oxford University Press, 2002), 3–4.

56 **"His body would become . . . At that point":** Sylvia Nasar, *A Beautiful Mind:*

The Life of Mathematical Genius and Nobel Laureate John Nash (New York: Simon & Schuster, 1994), 292.

56 **"Is it any wonder":** Edward Shorter, *A History of Psychiatry: From the Era of the Asylum to the Age of Prozac* (New York: John Wiley & Sons, 1997), 214; Norman S. Endler and Emmanuel Persad, *Electroconvulsive Therapy: The Myths and the Realities* (Toronto: Hans Huber Publishers, 1988), 5.

57–58 **"After 45 minutes of anxious":** Max Fink, "Autobiography of L.J. Meduna, Part Two," *Convulsive Therapy* 1, no. 2 (1985): 121–122.

58–59 **"Just before the convulsion":** Solomon Katzenelbogen, "Critical Appraisal of the 'Shock Therapies' in the Major Psychoses and Psychoneuroses III— Convulsive Therapy," *Psychiatry* 3 (1940): 412.

59–60 **Cerletti already had decided on dogs:** L. Bini, "Experimental Researches on Epileptic Attacks Induced by the Electric Current," *American Journal of Psychiatry* 94 (1938): 172–174.

60 **"This possibility we often discussed":** Ugo Cerletti, "Electroshock Therapy," *Journal of Clinical Experiments* 15, no. 3 (1954): 92.

61 **"caused all my doubts to vanish":** Cerletti, "Old and New Information," 90.

61 **"We agreed to have each session":** Accornero, "Eyewitness Account," 48.

61 **put a name to the new procedure:** Endler and Persad, *Electroconvulsive Therapy*, 20.

62 **gimmickry if not quackery:** Robert Whitaker, *Mad in America: Bad Science, Bad Medicine, and the Enduring Mistreatment of the Mentally Ill* (New York: Perseus Publishing, 2002), 41–81.

62–63 **reputation as snake pits . . . "Today's psychiatrists do not realize":** Shorter, *History of Psychiatry*, 190; Lothar B. Kalinowsky, "The Discoveries of Somatic Treatments in Psychiatry: Facts and Myths," *Comprehensive Psychiatry* 21, no. 6 (1980): 428.

63 **called the Johnny Appleseed of ECT:** Shorter, *History of Psychiatry*, 221.

63 **treatments at Rochester State Hospital:** Wellington W. Reynolds, "Electric Shock Treatment: Observations in 350 Cases," *Psychiatric Quarterly* 19 (1945): 322–333.

63–64 **"a rate four hundred times higher than today":** Matthew V. Rudorfer, Michael E. Henry, and Harold A. Sackeim, "Electroconvulsive Therapy," in *Psychiatry*, 2nd edition, ed. Allan Tasman, Jerald Kay, and Jeffery A. Lieberman (Hoboken, N.J.: 2003): 1884.

64–65 **"Patients were lined up":** Zigmond M. Lebensohn, "The History of Electroconvulsive Therapy in the United States and Its Place in American Psychiatry," *Comprehensive Psychiatry* 40, no. 3 (1999): 177.

65–66 **"A counterpane was pulled up to my neck":** Thelma G. Alper, "Case Reports: An Electric Shock Patient Tells His Story," *Journal of Abnormal and Social Psychology* 43 (1948): 205–207.

66 **U.S. Public Health Service survey:** Franklin G. Ebaugh, "A Review of the Drastic Shock Therapies in the Treatment of the Psychoses," *Annals of Internal Medicine* (March 1943): 279-296.

66 **McLean Hospital, in the Boston suburb:** W. Franklin Wood, letter to U.S. surgeon general transmitting report on shock therapies, March 14, 1942, McLean Hospital Archives.

66–67 **Stockton State Hospital, California's first insane asylum:** Joel Braslow, *Mental Ills and Bodily Cures: Psychiatric Treatment in the First Half of the Twentieth Century* (Berkeley: University of California Press, 1997), 100–101.

67 **"about nine-tenths of the mental hospitals":** Lucy Freeman, "Shock Treatment Held Not Enough," *New York Times,* April 14, 1949; "Gains Made in Help to Schizophrenics," *New York Times,* May 11, 1949, p. 8.

67 **It was tried with . . . homosexuality:** John A.P. Millet and Eric P. Mosse, "On Certain Psychological Aspects of Electroshock Therapy," *Psychosomatic Medicine* 6 (1944): 226–236.

68 **"diagnosis mattered little in doctors' decisions":** Braslow, *Mental Ills and Bodily Cures,* 101.

68–69 **Their first choice, curare:** www.botgard.ucla.edu/html/botanytexbooks/economicbotany/Curare; Shorter, *History of Psychiatry,* 223.

69 **Kalinowsky termed "unpleasant incidents":** Lothar B. Kalinowsky and Paul H. Hoch, *Shock Treatments and Other Somatic Procedures in Psychiatry* (New York: Grune & Stratton, 1946), 150.

70 **issues that would nearly kill the treatment:** Louis Lowinger and James H. Huddleson, "Complications in Electric Shock Therapy," *American Journal of Psychiatry* 102 (1946): 594–598; "Shock Treatment 'Ugly' to Pioneer," *New York Times,* April 24, 1959, p. 25.

71 **"pre-science" period:** Author interviews with Dr. Harold Sackeim, 2004 and 2005.

71 **"aiding the patients to forget":** Nolan D.C. Lewis, "The Present Status of Shock Therapy of Mental Disorders," *Bulletin of the New York Academy of Medicine* (1943): 236.

71–72 **"The first time I witnessed" . . . "a high percentage":** Zigmond M. Lebensohn, "Electroconvulsive Therapy: Psychiatry's Villain or Hero?," *American Journal of Social Psychiatry* 4, no. 4 (1984): 40; Abraham Myerson, "Borderline Cases Treated by Electric Shock," *American Journal of Psychiatry* 100 (1943): 355.

Chapter 6. In and Out of the Cuckoo's Nest

89–90 **a "device that might be said":** Ken Kesey, *One Flew Over the Cuckoo's Nest* (New York: Viking Press, 1962), 62, 245.

90 **Kesey's book was hailed:** Martin Levin, "A Reader's Report," *New York Times,* February 4, 1962, 214; "Life in the Loony Bin," *Time,* February 16, 1962, 90; *One Flew Over the Cuckoo's Nest,* 1975, directed by Milos Forman, Fantasy Films.

91 **"a clever little procedure":** Kesey, *Cuckoo's Nest,* 62.

92 **Other applications:** Robert E. Peck, *The Miracle of Shock Treatment* (Jericho, N.Y.: Exposition Press, 1974), 23; "Notes on Science: Stammering Cured by Electric Shock," *New York Times,* February 29, 1948, p. E11.

92–93 **"The evidence is conflicting":** "Shock Therapy," Group for the Advancement of Psychiatry, Report No. 1, September 15, 1947.

93 **"The field of psychiatry":** Author interview with Dr. Matthew Rudorfer, 2005.

93 **too many treatments:** "States' Rights vs. Victims' Rights," *New York Times,* May 8, 1977, 146; Bernard C. Glueck Jr., Harry Reiss, and Louis E. Bernard, "Regressive Electric Shock Therapy: Preliminary Report on 100 Cases," *Psychiatric Quarterly* 31, no. 1 (1957): 117–136.; Albert Rabin, "Patients Who Received More Than One Hundred Electric Shock Treatments," *Journal of Personality* 17 (1948): 42–47.

93–94 **REST treatment:** Glueck, Reiss, and Bernard, "Regressive Electric Shock Therapy," 117–136; "Electroconvulsive Therapy: National Institutes of Health Consensus Development Conference Statement" (1985): 1–23.

94–95 **Therapy as punishment:** William C. Ruffin, J. T. Monroe, and Gordon E. Rader, "Attitudes of Auxiliary Personnel Administering Electroconvulsive and Insulin Coma Treatment: A Comparative Study," *Journal of Nervous and Mental Disease* 131 (1960): 243; Dr. Peter G. Cranford, *But for the Grace of God: Milledgeville! The Inside Story of the World's Largest Insane Asylum* (Augusta, Ga.: Grand Pyramid Press, 1981), 108, 159.

95 **the experience at Stockton State Hospital:** Braslow, *Mental Ills and Bodily Cures* (Berkeley: University of California Press, 1997), 104.

95 **arrogant researcher or a pioneering healer:** Cerletti, "Electroshock Therapy," 205.

96 **"Except for the minority who yelled":** Ellen Field, *The White Shirts* (M. E. Redfield Publishers, 1964), 5, 7.

96 **In a moment of even greater candor:** Ugo Cerletti, "Electroshock Therapy," *Journal of Clinical Experiments* 15, no. 3 (1954): 193–194; Abram E. Bennett, "Evaluation of Progress in Established Physiochemical Treatments in Neuropsychiatry," *Diseases of the Nervous System* 7 (1949): 195–205.

97 **"forced electroshock":** Robert Whitaker, *Mad in America* (New York: Perseus Printing, 2002), 105.

97 **an experiment at Bellevue:** Lauretta Bender, "One Hundred Cases of Childhood Schizophrenia Treated with Electric Shock," *Transactions of the American Neurological Association* 72 (1947): 165–169.

97 **Rockland State Hospital:** E. R. Clardy and Elizabeth M. Rumpf, "The Effect of Electric Shock Treatment on Children Having Schizophrenic Manifestations," *Psychiatric Quarterly* 28, no. 4 (1954): 616–623.

98 **Chabasinski cannot remember details:** Author interview with Ted Chabasinski, 2005; Leonard Roy Frank, ed., *The History of Shock Treatment* (San Francisco: self-published by Frank, 1978).

98 **Bender went on to give:** Lauretta Bender, "The Development of a Schizophrenic Child Treated with Electric Convulsions at Three Years of Age," in *Emotional Problems of Early Childhood,* ed. Gerald Kaplan (New York: Basic Books, 1955), 407–430; Lauretta Bender, "Theory and Treatment of Childhood Schizophrenia," *Acta Paedopsychiatrica* 34 (1968): 298–307.

99 **electroshock's use in real torture:** Leonard S. Rubenstein, "The C.I.A. and the Evil Doctor," *New York Times,* November 7, 1988, p. A-19; Zigmond M. Lebensohn, "The History of Electroconvulsive Therapy in the United States and Its Place in American Psychiatry," *Comprehensive Psychiatry* 40, no. 3 (1999): 178.

101 **"as scientific as sticking one's head":** Citizens Commission on Human Rights Web site: http://www.cchr.org/index.cfm/6636.

101 **Scientology and its offshoots:** Citizens Commission on Human Rights, "Harming Artists: Psychiatry Ruins Creativity: Report and Recommendations on Psychiatry Assaulting the Arts," 19–20; L. Ron Hubbard, *Dianetics: The Modern Science of Mental Health* (New York: Hermitage House, 1950), 151.

101–102 **"our lives have been diminished":** Author interview with Leonard Roy Frank, 2005.

102 **"both cause brain tissue damage":** Peter Roger Breggin, *Electroshock: Its Brain-Disabling Effects* (New York: Springer Publishing Company, 1979), 198.

103–104 **A pair of UCLA doctors:** Barry Alan Kramer, "Use of ECT in California Revisited: 1984–1994," *Journal of ECT* 15, no. 4 (1999): 245–251; Peter Roy-Byrne and Robert H. Gerner, "Legal Restrictions on the Use of ECT in California: Clinical Impact on the Incompetent Patient," *Journal of Clinical Psychiatry* 42, no. 8 (1981): 300–303.

104 **"imagine . . . having a relative":** "States' Rights vs. Victims' Rights," *New York Times,* May 8, 1977, p. 146.

104 **While the number of patients:** Dr. Steven P. Shon, medical director for be-

havioral health, Texas Department of State Health Services, e-mail to author, 2005.

105 **"The classification of ECT":** Donald Kennedy, FDA commissioner, letter to Peter Sterling at the University of Pennsylvania, February 15, 1979, U.S. Food and Drug Administration Public Document Room, File 78N-1103.

105–106 **"There is in the minds of some people":** Christopher Lydon, "Eagleton Tells of Shock Therapy on Two Occasions," *New York Times,* July 26, 1972, p. 1.

106 **In Germany, researchers:** H. Lauter and H. Sauer, "Electroconvulsive Therapy: A German Perspective," *Convulsive Therapy* 3, no. 3 (1987): 207–208.

106 **Asked in 2005:** Author e-mail from Senator Thomas Eagleton, 2005.

107 **treatment today in Italy:** Psychoanalytic Institute for Social Research, "Ethical Aspects of Coercive Supervision and/or Treatment of Uncooperative Psychiatric Patients in the Community," Rome, Italy (1994); "Electroconvulsive Therapy Is Restricted in Italy," *The Lancet* 353 (1999): 993.

108–109 **"The wild, screaming, unapproachable patient":** Bliss Forbush, *The Sheppard & Enoch Pratt Hospital, 1853–1970: A History* (Philadelphia: J.B. Lippincott Company, 1971).

109–110 **ECT had no such benefactors:** Robin Nicol (president, Mecta Corporation), e-mail to author, 2005—Mecta and Somatics are the two U.S.-based ECT device makers; Marcia Angell, "The Truth About the Drug Companies," *New York Review of Books* 51, no. 12 (2004).

110 **"ECT is not profitable":** Keith Russell Ablow, *To Wrestle with Demons: A Psychiatrist Struggles to Understand His Patients and Himself* (New York: Carroll & Graf Publishers, Inc., 1992), 31.

111 **ECT's silver-screen debut:** *The Snake Pit,* 1948, Twentieth Century Fox Film Corp.

112 **The next movie, *Fear Strikes Out*:** *Fear Strikes Out,* 1956, Paramount Pictures.

113 **Two Australian psychiatrists:** Garry Walter and Andrew McDonald, "About to Have ECT? Fine, but Don't Watch It in the Movies: The Sorry Portrayal of ECT in Film," *Psychiatric Times* 21, no. 7 (2004).

113–114 **survey of workers in Ireland . . . poll of University of Arkansas medical:** Brian O'Shea and Aidan McGennis, "ECT: Lay Attitudes and Experiences— A Pilot Study," *British Medical Journal* 76, no. 1 (1983): 40–43; Jeffrey L. Clothier, Thomas Freeman, and Lisa Snow, "Medical Student Attitudes and Knowledge About ECT," *Journal of ECT* 17, no. 2 (2001): 99–101.

114 **Duke University study:** Y. Pritham Raj, "Medicine, Myths, and the Movies," *Post Graduate Medicine* 113, no. 6 (2003).

114 **"Kill Your Sons":** http://www.lyricsfreak.com/l/lou-reed/85253.html.

115 **"I had been subjected":** Gene Tierney with Mickey Herskowitz, *Self-Portrait* (New York: Wyden Books, 1979), 7, 202–203.

115 **"Then something bent down" . . . "I was given the new":** Sylvia Plath, *The Bell Jar* (New York: Alfred A. Knopf, 1998), 136; Janet Frame, *Janet Frame: An Autobiography* (Auckland, New Zealand: Random Century, 1989), 213, 238.

116 **"What is the sense of ruining my head":** A. E. Hotchner, *Papa Hemingway: A Personal Memoir* (New York: Random House, 1955), 279–280.

116 **He put the barrel into his mouth:** Jeffrey Meyers, *Hemingway: A Biography* (New York: Da Capo Press, 1999), 561.

116 **"it was on the first day" . . . had been talking about suicide:** CNN.Com/ specials/books/1999/hemingway/stories/biography/part3; Meyers, *Hemingway,* 561.

117 **"The big problem was that instead":** Author interview with A. E. Hotchner, 2005.

Chapter 8. Body of Evidence

127–128 **"At Washington University, where I trained":** Author interviews with and e-mails from Dr. Stephen Dinwiddie, 2004 and 2005.

128–129 **"We got him out of there":** Author interview with and e-mails from June Judge, 2005 and 2006.

130–131 **researchers at the Illinois State Psychiatric Institute . . . a 1997 study in Germany:** Philip G. Janicak et al., "Efficacy of ECT: A Meta-Analysis," *American Journal of Psychiatry* 142 (1985): 297–302; H. W. Folkerts et al., "Electroconvulsive Therapy vs. Paroxetine in Treatment-Resistant Depression—A Randomized Study," *Acta Psychiatrica Scandinavica* 96 (1997): 334.

132 **feeling more vital:** W. Vaughn McCall et al., "Health-Related Quality of Life Following ECT in a Large Community Sample," *Journal of Affective Disorders* 90 (2006): 269–274.

132 **"No controlled study" . . . "All considerations about ECT":** U.S. Department of Health and Human Services, "Mental Health: A Report of the Surgeon General" (1999), 258; "Electroconvulsive Therapy: National Institutes of Health Consensus Development Conference Statement" (1985): 1–23; Richard M. Glass, "Electroconvulsive Therapy: Time to Bring It Out of the Shadows," *Journal of the American Medical Association* 285, no. 10 (2001): 1346–1348.

132–133 **Eileen D. White was the sort of patient:** Author interviews with and e-mails from Eileen White, Dr. Thomas Jewitt, and Frederick Magnavito, 2005.

134 **"I got belted by electricity":** Author interview with Thomas Fitzgerald, 2005.

135 **a 1988 study comparing ECT head-to-head with lithium:** J. G. Small et al., "Electroconvulsive Treatment Compared with Lithium in the Management of Manic States," *Archives of General Psychiatry* 45, no. 8 (1988): 727–732.

135 **"Manic depression for me":** Andy Behrman, *Electroboy: A Memoir of Mania* (New York: Random House, 2002), xxi; author interview with Behrman, 2005.

135–136 **"five years of stability":** Author interview with Paul Cumming, 2005.

136 **"like a Stepford wife":** Author interview with Steve L., 2004.

137 **electroshock as an anticonvulsant therapy:** R. E. Hemphill, "The Treatment of Mental Disorders by Electrically Induced Convulsions," *Journal of Mental Sciences* 87 (1941): 256–275; Lothar B. Kalinowsky and Paul H. Hoch, *Shock Treatments and Other Somatic Procedures in Psychiatry* (New York: Grune & Stratton, 1946), 187; author interviews with Dr. Harold Sackeim and Dr. Sarah Lisanby, 2004 and 2005; C. P. Freeman, ed., *The ECT Handbook: The Second Report of the Royal College of Psychiatrists' Special Committee on ECT,* Council Report CR39 (1995), 15–16.

137–138 **"being trapped in a personal hell":** Author interview with and e-mails from Nancy Kopans, 2005.

138 **study by researchers in the Netherlands:** Jeroen A. van Waarde, Joost J. Stolker, and Rose C. van der Mast, "ECT in Mental Retardation: A Review," *Journal of ECT* 17, no. 4 (2001): 236–243.

139 **"I was, in fact, completely disabled":** Sherwin B. Nuland, *Lost in America: A Journey with My Father* (New York: Alfred A. Knopf, 2003), 4–7.

140 **That study, published in 2005:** Charles H. Kellner et al., "Relief of Expressed Suicidal Intent by ECT: A Consortium for Research in ECT Study," *American Journal of Psychiatry* 162 (2005): 5, 977–982.

140 **For each suicide a patient attempts:** Maria A. Oquendo et al., "Adequacy of Antidepressant Treatment After Discharge and the Occurrence of Suicidal Acts in Major Depression: A Prospective Study," *American Journal of Psychiatry* 159, no. 10 (2002): 1746–1751.

141 **"I took my shoelaces":** Author interview with Leslie Sladek-Sobczak, 2005.

141–142 **"I stopped counting":** Author interview with Carolyn, 2004.

142–143 **Studies on ECT and the elderly:** James D. Tew et al., "Acute Efficacy of ECT in the Treatment of Major Depression in the Old-Old," *American Journal of Psychiatry* 156, no. 12 (December 1999); American Psychiatric Association, *The Practice of Electroconvulsive Therapy: Recommendations for Treatment, Training, and Privileging,* 2nd ed. (Washington, D.C.: American Psychiatric Association, 2001), 43; Freeman, *The ECT Handbook,* 17; U.S. DHHS "Mental Health: A Report of the Surgeon General," 355.

144 **Yet the studies that have been run:** Joseph M. Rey and Garry Walter, "Half

a Century of ECT Use in Young People," *American Journal of Psychiatry* 154, no. 5 (1997): 595–602.

144 **In Paris, 60 percent . . . In Australia, 86 percent:** Olivier Taieb et al., "Electroconvulsive Therapy in Adolescents with Mood Disorder: Patients' and Parents' Attitudes," *Psychiatry Research* 104 (2001): 183–190; Garry Walter, Karryn Koster, and Joseph M. Rey, "Views About Treatment Among Parents of Adolescents Who Received Electroconvulsive Therapy," *Psychiatric Services* 50, no. 5 (1999): 701–702.

144 **multiyear investigation of the treatment:** "Practice Parameter for Use of Electroconvulsive Therapy with Adolescents," AACAP Official Action, *Journal of the American Academy of Child and Adolescent Psychiatry* 43, no. 12 (2004): 1521–1539.

144–145 **Alisson Wood is glad:** Author interview with Alisson Wood, 2005.

145 **ECT use during pregnancy:** Laura J. Miller, "Use of Electroconvulsive Therapy During Pregnancy," *Hospital and Community Psychiatry* 45, no. 5 (1994): 444–450.

145–146 **Declining use with schizophrenia:** James W. Thompson, Richard D. Weiner, and C. Patrick Myers, "Use of ECT in the United States in 1975, 1980, and 1986," *American Journal of Psychiatry* 151 (1994): 1657–1661.

146 **hard look at the use of ECT with schizophrenia:** Freeman, *The ECT Handbook,* 8–10; American Psychiatric Association, *Practice of Electroconvulsive Therapy,* 15–19; Matthew V. Rudorfer, Michael E. Henry, and Harold A. Sackeim, "Electroconvulsive Therapy," in *Psychiatry,* 2nd ed., ed. Allan Tasman et al. (Hoboken, N.J.: John Wiley & Sons, 2003), 1873–1874.

147 **"The hallucinations went away":** Author interview with Valerie, 2005.

147 **doctors in the community:** Richard C. Hermann et al., "Diagnoses of Patients Treated with ECT," *Psychiatric Services* 50, no. 8 (1999): 1059–1065; NIH Panel on Depression in Late Life, 1018–1024; Joan Prudic et al., "Effectiveness of Electroconvulsive Therapy in Community Settings," *Biological Psychiatry* 55, no. 2 (2004): 301–312.

148 **Studies on drug-resistant patients:** Joan Prudic et al., "Resistance to Antidepressant Medications and Short-Term Clinical Response to ECT," *American Journal of Psychiatry* 153, no. 8 (1996): 985–992; American Psychiatric Association, *Practice of Electroconvulsive Therapy,* 7–8.

149 **lithium together with the antidepressant nortriptyline:** Harold A. Sackeim et al., "Continuation Pharmacotherapy in the Prevention of Relapse Following Electroconvulsive Therapy: A Randomized Control Trial," *Journal of the American Medical Association* 285, no. 10 (2001): 1299–1307.

150 **More rigorous tests are under way:** Author interview with Dr. Charles Kellner, 2005.

150 **"The ECT treatments":** Author interview with Dr. Herbert Fox, 2004.

150 **"living in a fog":** Author interview with Christina Heath, 2005.

151 **"When many of the leading ECT practitioners":** Richard Abrams, *Electroconvulsive Therapy,* 4th ed. (New York: Oxford University Press, 2002), 8–9.

152 **For others the issue with psychotropics:** E-mail to author from Dr. Jerry Rosenbaum, 2005.

152 **plummeting from a high of 559,000:** Edward Shorter, *A History of Psychiatry* (New York: John Wiley & Sons, 1997), 280.

153 **"It was love at first sight":** Author interviews with Dr. Charles Welch, 2004 and 2005.

153–154 **"for people involved with ECT":** Author interviews with Sackeim.

154 **first rather than last treatment:** American Psychiatric Association, *Practice of Electroconvulsive Therapy,* 6–7.

155 **"I wonder what would have happened":** Author interview with Dr. Leon Rosenberg, 2005.

Chapter 10. Complications and Controversies

164–165 **Now comes Anne Donahue:** Anne B. Donahue, "Electroconvulsive Therapy and Memory Loss: A Personal Journey," *Journal of ECT* 16, no. 2 (2000): 133–143; author interviews with and e-mails from Anne Donahue, 2005.

166 **"a personal conviction":** Richard Abrams, *Electroconvulsive Therapy,* 4th ed. (New York: Oxford University Press, 2002), 200.

166 **"I agree with Anne's assessment":** Dr. Deborah N. Black, Green Mountain Neurology, written office notes after checkup of Anne Donahue on June 25, 2003.

167 **"I was being told":** Author interviews with and e-mails from Donahue.

167 **serious medical injuries:** "Electroconvulsive Therapy: National Institutes of Health Consensus Development Conference Statement" (1985): 1–23.

167 **The death rate in ECT's:** "Electroconvulsive Therapy: National Institutes of Health Consensus Development Conference Statement" (1985): 1–23.

168 **"mental symptoms":** Lothar B. Kalinowsky and Paul H. Hoch, *Shock Treatments and Other Somatic Procedures in Psychiatry* (New York: Grune & Stratton, 1950), 131–132.

168 **Recollections most likely to disappear:** Sarah H. Lisanby et al., "The Effects of Electroconvulsive Therapy on Memory of Autobiographical and Public Events," *Archives of General Psychiatry* 57 (2000): 581–590; NIH Consensus Development Conference, 1–23.

169 **new study from Columbia University:** Harold A. Sackeim et al., "The Cognitive Effects of Electroconvulsive Therapy in Community Settings," [awaiting publication].

169–170 **ask large numbers of patients:** C.P.L. Freeman and R. E. Kendell, "ECT: I. Patients' Experiences and Attitudes," *British Journal of Psychiatry* 137 (1980): 8–16; Diana Rose et al., "Patients' Perspectives on Electroconvulsive Therapy: Systematic Review," *British Medical Journal* 326 (2003): 1363–1367; Eliza A. Coleman et al., "Subjective Memory Complaints Prior to and Following Electroconvulsive Therapy," *Biological Psychiatry* 39 (1996): 346–356.

170 **big mental health advocacy groups:** Official positions provided by the Depression and Bipolar Support Alliance, National Mental Health Association, and National Alliance on Mental Illness.

170–171 **"tend not to stay in our practices":** Author interviews with Dr. Charles Welch.

171 **"Everyone always asks"** . . . **"a little bit of short-term memory loss":** Author interviews with Christina Heath and Donna Orrin, 2005.

171 **"explicit, short-term memory":** Jonathan Cott, *On the Sea of Memory* (New York: Random House, 2005), 8–9.

172 **"My mother left":** Author interview with Karren S. Jones, 2005.

172–173 **"as a shield against anxiety":** William Styron, *Darkness Visible: A Memoir of Madness* (New York: Vintage Books, 1992), 43; author interview with William Styron and Rose Styron, 2005.

173 **belief that lost memories:** John Friedberg, *Shock Treatment Is Not Good for Your Brain* (San Francisco: Glide, 1976); Peter Roger Breggin, *Electroshock: Its Brain-Disabling Effects* (New York: Springer Publishing Company, 1979); Breggin, "Electroshock: Scientific, Ethical, and Political Issues," *International Journal of Risk & Safety in Medicine* 11 (1998): 5–40; Peter Sterling, "ECT Damage Is Easy to Find If You Look for It," *Nature* 403 (2000): 242; Testimony of Leonard Roy Frank at a Public Hearing Before the Mental Health Committee of the New York State Assembly, May 18, 2001.

173–174 **The case *for* brain damage:** B. J. Alpers and J. Hughes, "The Brain Changes in Electrically Induced Convulsions in the Human," *Journal of Neuropathology and Experimental Neurology* 1 (1942): 173–180; Armando Ferraro and Leon Roizin, "Cerebral Morphologic Changes in Monkeys Subjected to a Large Number of Electrically Induced Convulsions (32–100)," *American Journal of Psychiatry* 106, no. 4 (1949): 278–284; Lothar B. Kalinowsky, "Organic Psychotic Syndromes Occurring During Electric Convulsive Therapy," *Archives of Neurology and Psychiatry* 53 (1945): 269–273.

174 **"the damaging effects of ECT":** John Friedberg, "Shock Treatment, Brain Damage, and Memory Loss: A Neurological Perspective," *American Journal of Psychiatry* 134, no. 9 (1977): 1011.

175 **University of Louisville study:** Steven Lippmann et al., "1,250 Electroconvul-

sive Treatments without Evidence of Brain Injury," *British Journal of Psychiatry* 147 (1985): 203–204.

175–176 **The case *against* brain damage:** Richard D. Weiner, "Does Electroconvulsive Therapy Cause Brain Damage?" *Behavioral and Brain Sciences* 7 (1984): 1; Dr. C. Edward Coffey, ed., *The Clinical Science of Electroconvulsive Therapy* (Washington, D.C.: American Psychiatric Press, Inc., 1993), 88; Andrew J. Dwork et al., "Absence of Histological Lesions in Primate Models of ECT and Magnetic Seizure Therapy, Brief Report," *American Journal of Psychiatry* 161, no. 3 (2004): 576–578; author interviews with Dr. Sarah Lisanby (2004 and 2005).

176 **"Forced" shock:** The most recent annual ECT reports filed by Illinois, California, and Texas; author interview with David Oaks, 2005; http://www.mindfreedom.org.

177 **"nobody likes to do involuntary treatment":** Author interview with and e-mail from Dr. Benjamin Liptzin, 2005.

177 **Asking for consent:** Abram E. Bennett, "Evaluation of Progress in Established Physiochemical Treatments in Neuropsychiatry," *Diseases of the Nervous System* 7 (July 1949): 204; Superior Court of the State of California for the County of Santa Barbara, Case No. 1069713, *Atze Akkerman and Elizabeth Akkerman vs Joseph Johnson, Santa Barbara Cottage Hospital et al.,* January 2, 2005, decision; Vermont Department of Developmental and Mental Health Services, Informed Consent Package for Electroconvulsive Therapy, revised 10/01 and 11/04; Dartmouth–Hitchcock Medical Center, "Electroconvulsive Therapy" videotape, Department of Psychiatry.

178 **Authors of a French review . . . In a British study:** Olivier Taieb et al., "Electroconvulsive Therapy in Adolescents with Mood Disorder: Patient's and Parents' Attitudes," *Psychiatry Research* 104, no. 2 (2001): 183–190; S. M. Benbow, "Patients' Views on Electroconvulsive Therapy on Completion of a Course of Treatment," *Convulsive Therapy* 4, no. 2 (1988): 146–152.

178–179 **"I should have asked":** Author interview with and e-mails from Sister Barbara.

179 **as the Vermont concurrence form recommends:** Vermont, Informed Consent Package; Donahue, "A Personal Journey," 133–143.

179–180 **A favorite target of critics:** Author e-mail from Dr. Richard Abrams, June 15, 2005; Abrams, *Electroconvulsive Therapy,* 10; author interview with David Mirkovich of Somatics, 2005.

180 **collaborated with one or both ECT device makers:** Author interview with Robin Nicol of Mecta Corporation, 2005.

181 **"a lie-detector-like device":** Thomas M. Burton, "Medical Flap: Anti-

Depression Drug of Eli Lilly Loses Sales After Attack by Sect," *Wall Street Journal,* April 19, 1991.

181 **"In shock cases, such as electric shock":** L. Ron Hubbard, *Dianetics: The Modern Science of Mental Health* (Los Angeles: Bridge Publications, 1950), 490; Citizens Commission on Human Rights Web site: http://www.cchr.org/index.cfm.

181 **CCHR says on its Web site:** http://www.cchr.org/index.cfm.

182 **"The focus on Scientology":** Author interview with and e-mail from Frank, 2005.

183 **"taking patients who are the sickest":** Author interviews with Dr. Harold Sackeim (2004 and 2005).

184 **Newer findings by the Columbia scientists:** Harold A. Sackeim et al., "A Prospective, Randomized, Double-Blind Comparison of Bilateral and Right Unilateral Electroconvulsive Therapy at Different Stimulus Intensities," *Archives of General Psychiatry* 57, no. 5 (2000): 425–434; Sackeim et al., "Cognitive Effects of Electroconvulsive Therapy."

184–185 **Bilateral v unilateral ECT:** Author interviews with Dr. Charles Kellner (2005), Dr. Max Fink (2004 and 2005), Dr. Richard Weiner (2005), and Sackeim; American Psychiatric Association, *Practice of Electroconvulsive Therapy,* 153.

185 **A sine wave is the kind of current:** American Psychiatric Association, *Practice of Electroconvulsive Therapy* (Washington, D.C.: American Psychiatric Association, 1990), 141; author interviews with Sackeim.

185–186 **how to decide on the right dose:** American Psychiatric Association, *Practice of Electroconvulsive Therapy,* 158–161.

186 **The last debate on technique is over frequency:** Ibid., 174–175.

187 **not everyone pays attention:** Andy Farah and W. Vaughn McCall, "Electroconvulsive Therapy Stimulus Dosing: A Survey of Contemporary Practices," *Convulsive Therapy* 9, no. 2 (1993): 90–94; Joan Prudic, Mark Olfson, and Harold A. Sackeim. "Electro-Convulsive Therapy Practices in the Community," *Psychological Medicine* 31, no. 5 (2001): 929–934; author interviews with Lisanby.

187 **debate over ECT technique:** Author interviews with Dr. W. Vaughn McCall (2005), an ECT patient from Boston who asked that his name not be used, and Pierre.

188 **"I honestly believe":** Author interview with Susan Kadis, 2005.

188 **"zoned out and really having a hard time":** Author interview with Steven A. Katz, 2005.

189 **Anne Donahue wants to build:** Donahue, "A Personal Journey," 133–143; author interviews with and e-mails from Donahue.

Chapter 12. The Mystery of How and Why

196 **"The black box still is pretty black":** Author interview with Dr. Thomas Neylan, 2005.

196–197 **"Not knowing how ECT works":** Keith Russell Ablow, *To Wrestle with Demons* (New York: Carroll & Graf Publishers, 1992), 29.

197 **"We don't know why":** Author interview with Orrin.

197–198 **ECT might produce damage:** Franklin G. Ebaugh, Clarke H. Barnacle, and Karl T. Neubuerger, "Fatalities Following Electric Convulsive Therapy: A Report of 2 Cases with Autopsy Findings," *Archives of Neurology and Psychiatry* 49, no. 107 (1943): 39; Abram E. Bennett, "Evaluation of Progress in Established Physiochemical Treatments in Neuropsychiatry," *Diseases of the Nervous System* 7 (July 1949): 197; Max Fink, "Effect of Anticholinergic Agent, Diethazine, on EEG and Behavior: Significance for Theory of Convulsive Therapy," *Archives of Neurology and Psychiatry* 80 (1958): 384.

198 **Doctors drew on psychoanalytic reasoning:** Nolan D.C. Lewis, "The Present Status of Shock Therapy of Mental Disorders," *Bulletin of the New York Academy of Medicine* (April 1943): 236; Herman Selinski, "The Selective Use of Electro-Shock Therapy as an Adjuvant to Psychotherapy," *Bulletin of the New York Academy of Medicine* (1943): 250–251.

198–199 **So many were the early interpretations:** Major Hirsch L. Gordon, "Fifty Shock Therapy Theories," *Military Surgeon* 103 (1948): 397–401.

199 **"It is extremely probable":** Ugo Cerletti, "Electroshock Therapy," *Journal of Clinical Experiments* 15, no. 3 (September 1954): 204.

199 **"the exact mechanism":** Joel Braslow, *Mental Ills and Bodily Cures* (Berkeley: University of California Press, 1997), 103–104.

200 **"We all may have the brain structure":** Harold A. Sackeim, "The Case for ECT," *Psychology Today* 19, no. 6 (1985); author interviews with Dr. Harold Sackeim (2004 and 2005).

200 **"We know a lot about what ECT":** Author interviews with Dr. Sarah Lisanby (2004 and 2005).

201 **The more dispersion the better:** Richard Abrams, *Electroconvulsive Therapy*, 4th ed. (New York: Oxford University Press, 2002), 218–222.

201 **"Why does the patient get better?":** Author interviews with Dr. Max Fink (2004 and 2005). Fink, "Electroshock Revisited," *American Scientist* 88, no. 2 (2000): 162.

202 **remains unknown and perhaps unknowable:** Author interview with Dr. Descartes Li, 2005; Abrams, *Electroconvulsive Therapy*, 223.

202–203 **patient theories on how ECT works:** "New Sparks over Electroshock,"

Time, February 26, 2001, 60–62; Sherwin Nuland, *Lost in America* (New York: Alfred A. Knopf, 2003), 7–8; Andy Behrman, *Electroboy: A Memoir of Mania* (New York: Random House, 2002), 226, 232.

203 **"cut all the connections":** Robert E. Peck, *The Miracle of Shock Treatment* (Jericho, N.Y.: Exposition Press, 1974), 31.

203 **"How we trick the brain":** Author e-mails from and interviews with Dr. Charles Welch (2004 and 2005).

205 **"If you want to fill this glass":** Author interviews with and e-mails from Dr. Alvaro Pascual-Leone, 2005.

206 **"a barrage of different medications":** Author interview with Mike Henry, 2005.

207 **"staged approach":** Author interviews with Lisanby.

208 **studies on bifrontal ECT:** F. J. Letemendia, N. J. Delva, and M. Rodenburg et al., "Therapeutic Advantage of Bifrontal Electrode Placement in ECT," *Psychological Medicine* 23 (1993): 349–360; Samuel H. Bailine et al., "Comparison of Bifrontal and Bitemporal ECT for Major Depression," *American Journal of Psychiatry* 157 (2000): 121–123.

208 **who feels the new technologies:** Author interviews with Fink.

209 **"the problem with drugs":** Author interviews with Sackeim.

BIBLIOGRAPHY

Ablow, Keith Russell. *To Wrestle with Demons: A Psychiatrist Struggles to Understand His Patients and Himself.* New York: Carroll & Graf Publishers, 1992.

Abrams, Richard. *Electroconvulsive Therapy,* 4th ed. New York: Oxford University Press, 2002.

———. "The FDA Proposal to Reclassify ECT Devices." *Convulsive Therapy* 7, no. 1 (1991): 1–4.

———. "The Mortality Rate with ECT." *Convulsive Therapy* 13, no. 3 (1997): 125–127.

———. "'Safe, Effective and Widely Used' Electroconvulsive Therapy." Letter to editor, *New York Times,* November 25, 1982.

Abrams, Richard, Conrad M. Swartz, and Chandragupta Vedak. "Antidepressant Effects of High-Dose Right Unilateral Electroconvulsive Therapy." *Archives of General Psychiatry* 48, no. 8 (1991): 746–748.

———. "Antidepressant Effects of Right Versus Left Unilateral ECT and the Lateralization Theory of ECT Action." *American Journal of Psychiatry* 146, no. 9 (1989): 1190–1192.

Abrams, Richard, Michael Alan Taylor, and Jan Volavka. "ECT-Induced EEG Asymmetry and Therapeutic Response in Melancholia: Relation to Treatment Electrode Placement." *American Journal of Psychiatry* 144, no. 3 (1987): 327–329.

Abse, David Wilfred, and John A. Ewing. "Transference and Countertransference in

Bibliography

Somatic Therapies." *Journal of Nervous and Mental Disease* 123, no. 1 (January 1956): 32–40.

Accornero, Ferdinando. "An Eyewitness Account of the Discovery of Electroshock," *Convulsive Therapy* 4, no. 1 (1988): 40–49.

Aden et al. v. Younger, 57 Calif. 3d 662 (1976).

Aden, Gary C. "The International Psychiatric Association for the Advancement of Electrotherapy: A Brief History." *American Journal of Social Psychiatry* 4 (Fall 1984): 18–21.

Alper, Thelma G. "Case Reports: An Electric Shock Patient Tells His Story." *Journal of Abnormal and Social Psychology* 43 (1948): 201–210.

Alpers, B. J., and J. Hughes. "The Brain Changes in Electrically Induced Convulsions in the Human." *Journal of Neuropathology and Experimental Neurology* 1 (1942): 173–180.

Altman, Lawrence K. "Two Doctors, on Ethical Grounds, Are Silent on Eagleton's Case." *New York Times*, July 27, 1972.

American Psychiatric Association. "Electroconvulsive Therapy: Fact Sheet." October 1997.

———. *The Practice of Electroconvulsive Therapy: Recommendations for Treatment, Training, and Privileging*, Washington, D.C.: American Psychiatric Association, 1990.

———. *The Practice of Electroconvulsive Therapy: Recommendations for Treatment, Training, and Privileging*, 2nd ed. Washington, D.C.: American Psychiatric Association, 2001.

Andersson, J. E., and T. G. Bolwig. "Electroconvulsive Therapy in Denmark 1999: A Nation-Wide Questionnaire Study." *Ugeskr Laeger* 164, no. 26 (June 2002): 3449–3452.

Andrade, Chittaranjan, Alexander I. Nelson, and Max Fink. "ECT in the Management of Major Depression: Implications of Recent Research." *World Journal of Biological Psychiatry* 4, no. 3 (July 2003): 139–141.

Andrade, Chittaranjan, Nilesh Shah, and Prathap Tharyan. "The Dilemma of Unmodified ECT." *Journal of Clinical Psychiatry* 64, no. 10 (October 2003): 1147–1152.

Andre, Linda. "Lying for Fun and Profit: Information About Convulsive Therapy." Available at: http://www.ect.org. June 8, 2005.

Angel at My Table, An. Film. Directed by Jane Campion. Criterion, 1990.

Angell, Marcia. "The Truth About the Drug Companies." *New York Review of Books* 51, no. 12 (July 15, 2004).

Anonymous. "How I Owe My Life to ECT—By a Practicing Psychiatrist." *American Journal of Social Psychiatry* 4 (Fall 1984): 16–17.

"Anti-ECT Legislation in Texas." *Convulsive Therapy* 11, no. 2 (1995): 148–153.

Asnis, Gregory M., Max Fink, and Sue Saferstein. "ECT in Metropolitan New York

Hospitals: A Survey of Practice, 1975–1976." *American Journal of Psychiatry* 135, no. 4 (1978): 479–482.

Associated Press. "Psychiatric Tactics Target of Protest." *New York Times*, May 3, 1983.

Association for Convulsive Therapy. Survey of Members, 2005.

Avery, David, and George Winokur. "Mortality in Depressed Patients Treated with Electroconvulsive Therapy and Antidepressants." *Archives of General Psychiatry* 33, no. 9 (September 1976): 1029–1037.

———. "Suicide, Attempted Suicide, and Relapse Rates in Depression." *Archives of General Psychiatry* 35, no. 6 (1978): 749–753.

Babigian, Haroutun M., and Laurence B. Guttmacher. "Epidemiological Considerations in Electroconvulsive Therapy." *Archives of General Psychiatry* 41, no. 3 (1984): 246–253.

Bailine, Samuel H., Arthur Rifkin, Ernst Kayne, Jeffery A. Selzer, Jacques Vital-Herner, Marjorie Blicka, and Simcha Pollack. "Comparison of Bifrontal and Bitemporal ECT for Major Depression." *American Journal of Psychiatry* 157, no. 1 (2000): 121–123.

Balabanov, Antoaneta, and Andres M. Kanner. "Unrecognized and Untreated: Preventing and Treating Depression in Patients with Epilepsy." *Psychiatric Times* 23, no. 13 (November 1, 2004).

Baldwin, Steve, and Melissa Oxlad. *Electroshock and Minors: A Fifty-Year Review.* Westport, Conn.: Greenwood Press, 2000.

Barker, J. C., and A. A. Baker. "Deaths Associated with Electroplexy." *Journal of Mental Science* 105, no. 439 (1959): 339–348.

Baxter, Lewis R., Peter Roy-Byrne, Edward H. Liston, and Lynn Fairbanks. "The Experience of Electroconvulsive Therapy in the 1980s: A Prospective Study of the Knowledge, Opinions, and Experience of California Electroconvulsive Therapy Patients in the Berkeley Years." *Convulsive Therapy* 2, no. 3 (1986): 179–189.

Beam, Alex. *Gracefully Insane: The Rise and Fall of America's Premiere Mental Hospital.* New York: Public Affairs, 2001.

Beautiful Mind, A. Film. Directed by Ron Howard. Universal Pictures, 2001.

Behrman, Andy. *Electroboy: A Memoir of Mania.* New York: Random House, 2002.

———. "Electroboy: He Was Hooked Up, Switched On, Blissed Out." *New York Times Magazine,* January 24, 1999.

Benbow, S. M. "Patients' Views on Electroconvulsive Therapy on Completion of a Course of Treatment." *Convulsive Therapy* 4, no. 2 (1988): 146–152.

Bender, Lauretta. "The Development of a Schizophrenic Child Treated with Electric Convulsions at Three Years of Age." In *Emotional Problems of Early Childhood,* pp. 407–430. Edited by Gerald Kaplan. New York: Basic Books, 1955.

————."One Hundred Cases of Childhood Schizophrenia Treated with Electric Shock." *Transactions of the American Neurological Association* 72 (June 18, 1947): 165–169.

————. "Theory and Treatment of Childhood Schizophrenia." *Acta Paedopsychiatrica* 34 (1968): 298–307.

————. "Twenty Years of Clinical Research on Schizophrenic Children, with Special Reference to Those Under Six Years of Age." In *Emotional Problems of Early Childhood,* pp. 503–515. Edited by Gerald Kaplan. New York: Basic Books, 1955.

Bennett, Abram E. "Evaluation of Progress in Established Physiochemical Treatments in Neuropsychiatry." *Diseases of the Nervous System* 7 (July 1949): 195–205.

Bertagnolia, Mark W., and Carrie M. Borchardt. "Case Study: A Review of ECT for Children and Adolescents." *Journal of the American Academy of Child & Adolescent Psychiatry* 29, no. 2 (1990): 302–307.

Beverly Hillbillies, The. Film. Directed by Penelope Spheeris. Twentieth Century Fox, 1993.

Bidder, T. G., J. J. Strain, and L. Brunschwig. "Bilateral and Unilateral ECT: Follow-up Study and Critique." *American Journal of Psychiatry* 127, no. 6 (1970): 737–745.

Bielski, Vince. "Electroshock's Quiet Comeback." *San Francisco Bay Guardian,* April 18, 1990, pp.18–21.

Bini, L. "Experimental Researches on Epileptic Attacks Induced by the Electric Current." *American Journal of Psychiatry* 94 (1938): 172–174.

Birrer, Richard B., and Sathya P. Vemuri. "Depression in Later Life: A Diagnostic and Therapeutic Challenge." *American Family Physician* 69, no. 10 (May 15, 2004): 2375–2382.

Black, Deborah N. Written office notes from Dr. Deborah N. Black, Green Mountain Neurology, after checkup of Anne Donahue on June 25, 2003.

Black, Donald W., George Winokur, Emmanuel Mohandoss, Robert F. Woolson, and Amelia Nasrallah. "Does Treatment Influence Mortality in Depressives? A Follow-up of 1,076 Patients with Major Affective Disorders." *Annals of Clinical Psychiatry* 1 (1989): 165–173.

Blek, Libby, and Leslie Navran. "Somatic Therapy as Discussed by Psychotic Patients." *Journal of Abnormal Psychology* 50, no. 3 (May 1955): 394–400.

Bloch, Yuval, Yechiel Levcovitch, Aviva Mimouni Bloch, Shlomo Mendlovic, and Gideon Ratzoni. "Electroconvulsive Therapy in Adolescents: Similarities to and Differences from Adults." *Journal of the American Academy of Child & Adolescent Psychiatry* 40, no. 11 (November 2001): 1332–1336.

Bloch, Yuval, Gideon Ratzoni, Doli Sobol, Shlomo Mendlovic, and Gideon Ratzoni.

"Gender Differences in Electroconvulsive Therapy: A Retrospective Chart Review." *Journal of Affective Disorders* 84, no. 1 (January 2005): 99–102.

Boesky, Howard M. "Psychotherapy Can Help Depressions." *New York Times,* February 23, 1992.

Boodman, Sangra G. "Shock Therapy: It's Back." *Washington Post,* September 24, 1996, sec. Z, p. 14.

Boronow, John, Anne Stoline, and Steve S. Sharfstein. "Refusal of ECT by a Patient with Recurrent Depression, Psychosis, and Catatonia." *American Journal of Psychiatry* 154, no. 9 (1997): 1285–1291.

Boyer, L. Bryce. "Fantasies Concerning ECT." *Psychoanalytic Review* 39 (1952): 252–270.

Boyland, Laura S., Roger F. Haskett, Benoit H. Mulsant, Robert M. Greenberg, Joan Prudic, Kerith Spicknall, Sarah H. Lisanby, and Harold A. Sackeim. "Determinants of Seizure Threshold in ECT: Benzodiazepine Use, Anesthetic Dosage, and Other Factors." *Journal of ECT* 16, no. 1 (2000): 3–18.

Braslow, Joel. *Mental Ills and Bodily Cures: Psychiatric Treatment in the First Half of the Twentieth Century.* Berkeley: University of California Press, 1997.

Breggin, Peter Roger. *Electroshock: Its Brain-Disabling Effects.* New York: Springer Publishing Company, 1979.

———. "Electroshock: Scientific, Ethical, and Political Issues." *International Journal of Risk & Safety in Medicine* 11 (1998): 5–40.

———. *Toxic Psychiatry: Why Therapy, Empathy, and Love Must Replace the Drugs, Electroshock, and Biochemical Theories of the "New Psychiatry."* New York: St. Martin's Press, 1991.

Brodaty, Henry, Ian Hickie, Catherine Mason, and Leanne Prenter. "A Prospective Follow-up Study of ECT Outcome in Older Depressed Patients." *Journal of Affective Disorders* 60, no. 2 (2000): 101–111.

Brown, David. "At Psychiatry Meeting, Ex-Patients Protest Mental Health Treatment." *Washington Post,* May 4, 1992, sec. A, p. 6.

Brussel, James A., and Jacob Schneider. "The B.E.S.T. in the Treatment and Control of Chronically Disturbed Mental Patients—A Preliminary Report." *Psychology Quarterly* 25, no. 1 (January 1951): 55–64.

Burns, Veronica. "Goodbye, Darkness: A TV Host's Odyssey from Terrifying Depression to Renewed Peace of Mind." *People,* August 3, 1992.

Burt, Tal, Sarah H. Lisanby, and Harold A. Sackeim. "Neuropsychiatric Applications of TMS: A Meta Analysis." *International Journal of Neuropsychopharmacology* 5, no. 1 (March 2002): 73–103.

Burton, Thomas M. "Medical Flap: Anti-Depression Drug of Eli Lilly Loses Sales After Attack by Sect." *Wall Street Journal,* April 19, 1991, p. A-1.

• • •

Calev, Avraham, Elena Kochav-lev, Nurith Tubi, Doran Nigal, Shella Chazan, Baruch Shapira, and Bernard Lerer. "Change in Attitude Toward Electroconvulsive Therapy: Effects of Treatment, Time Since Treatment, and Severity of Depression." *Convulsive Therapy* 7, no. 3 (1991): 184–189.

Calev, Avraham, Doron Nigal, Baruch Shapira, Nurith Tubi, Shella Chazan, Yoram Ben-Yehuda, Sol Kugelmass, and Bernard Lerer. "Early and Long-Term Effects of Electroconvulsive Therapy and Depression on Memory and Other Cognitive Functions." *Journal of Nervous and Mental Disease* 179, no. 9 (1991): 526–533.

California Department of Mental Health. "Annual Report on Electroconvulsive Therapy in California," 1977–2002.

Calloway, S. P., R. J. Dolan, R. J. Jacoby, and R. Levy. "ECT and Cerebral Atrophy." *Acta Psychiatrica Scandanavia* 64, no. 5 (November 1981): 442–445.

Cameron, D. Ewen. "Production of Differential Amnesia as a Factor in the Treatment of Schizophrenia." *Comparative Psychiatry* 1 (February 1960): 26–34.

Cameron, Douglas G. "ECT: Sham Statistics, the Myth of Convulsive Therapy, and the Case for Consumer Misinformation." *Journal of Mind and Behavior* 15, nos. 1–2 (1994): 177–198.

Carney, Stuart, and John Geddes. "Electroconvulsive Therapy: Recent Recommendations Are Likely to Improve Standards and Uniformity of Use." *British Medical Journal* 326 (June 21, 2003): 1343–1344.

Casey, David A., and Mary Helen Davis. "Electroconvulsive Therapy in the Very Old." *General Hospital Psychiatry* 18, no. 6 (November 1996): 436–439.

Cauchon, Dennis. "Controversy and Questions: Shock Therapy." *USA Today*, December 6–7, 1995: 1; 4D.

Cerletti, Ugo. "Electroshock Therapy." *Journal of Clinical Experiments* 15, no. 3 (September 1954): 191–217.

———. "Old and New Information About Electroshock." *American Journal of Psychiatry* 107 (1950): 87–94.

Chanpattana, Worrawat, M. L. Somchai Chakrabhand, Wanchai Buppanharun, and Harold A. Sackeim. "Effects of Stimulus Intensity on the Efficacy of Bilateral ECT in Schizophrenia: A Preliminary Study." *Biological Psychiatry* 48, no. 3 (2000): 222–228.

Chanpattana, Worrawat, Kasuki Kojima, Barry Alan Kramer, Aim Intakorn, and Satoshi Sasaki. "ECT Practice in Japan." *Journal of ECT* 21, no. 1 (March 2005): 58.

Chanpattana, Worrawat, Girish Kunigiri, Barry Alan Kramer, and B. N. Gangadhar. "Survey of the Practice of Electroconvulsive Therapy in Teaching Hospitals in India." *Journal of ECT* 21, no. 2 (June 2005): 100–104.

Chistyakov, Andrei V., Boris Kaplan, Odil Rubicheck, Isabella Kreinin, Dani Koren,

Hava Hafner, Moshe Feinsod, and Ehud Klein. "Effect of Electroconvulsive Therapy on Cortical Excitability in Patients with Major Depression: A Transcranial Magnetic Stimulation Study." *Clinical Neurophysiology* 116, no. 2 (2005): 386–392.

Chongcheng, Xue, Xie Huansen, Ruan Qingchi, Cheng Yuande, and Luo Dingli. "Electric Acupuncture Convulsive Therapy." *Convulsive Therapy* 1, no. 4 (1985): 242–251.

Citizens Commission on Human Rights. "The Brutal Reality: Harmful Psychiatric 'Treatments.'"

———. "Creating Harm: The History of Electroshock."

———. "Harming Artists: Psychiatry Ruins Creativity," 1969.

———. http://www.cchr.org/.

Cizadlo, Beth C., and Wheaton, Allyson. "Case Study: ECT Treatment of a Young Girl with Catatonia." *Journal of the American Academy of Child & Adolescent Psychiatry* 34, no. 3 (March 1995): 332–335.

Clardy, E. R., and Elizabeth M. Rumpf. "The Effect of Electric Shock Treatment on Children Having Schizophrenic Manifestations." *Psychiatric Quarterly* 28, no. 4 (1954): 616–623.

"Clinical Trial of the Treatment of Depressive Illness: Report to the Medical Research Council by Its Clinical Psychiatry Committee." *British Medical Journal* 1 (April 3, 1965): 881–886.

Clothier, Jeffrey L., Thomas Freeman, and Lisa Snow. "Medical Student Attitudes and Knowledge About ECT." *Journal of ECT* 17, no. 2 (2001): 99–101.

CNN. http://www.cnn.com/SPECIALS/books/1999/hemingway/.

Coffey, C. Edward, ed. *The Clinical Science of Electroconvulsive Therapy.* Washington, D.C.: American Psychiatric Press, 1993.

Coffey, C. Edward, and Richard D. Weiner. "Electroconvulsive Therapy: An Update." *Hospital and Community Psychiatry* 41, no. 5 (May 1990): 515–521.

Cohen, David. "Electroconvulsive Treatment, Neurology and Psychiatry." *Ethical Human Sciences and Services* 3, no. 2 (2001): 127–129.

Cohen, David, Martine Flament, Pierre-Francois Dubos, and Michel Basquin. "Case Series: Cationic Syndrome in Young People." *Journal of the American Academy of Child & Adolescent Psychiatry* 38, no. 8 (August 1, 1999): 1040–1046.

Cohen, David, O. Taieb, Martine Flament, Sylvie Chevret, Philippe Fossati, Jean-Francois Allilaire, and Michel Basquin. "Absence of Cognitive Impairment at Long-Term Follow-up in Adolescents Treated with ECT for Severe Mood Disorder." *American Journal of Psychiatry* 157, no. 3 (2000): 460–462.

Cole, Catherine, and Robert Tobiansky. "Electroconvulsive Therapy: NICE Guidance May Deny Many Patients Treatment That They Might Benefit From." *British Medical Journal* 327 (September 13, 2003): 621.

Coleman, Eliza A., Harold A. Sackeim, Joan Prudic, D. P. Devanand, Martin C. McElhiney, and Bobba J. Moody. "Subjective Memory Complaints Prior to and Following Electroconvulsive Therapy." *Biological Psychiatry* 39 (1996): 346–356.

Coleman, Lee. *The Reign of Error: A Startling Exposé of Psychiatry's Misrule in the Courts, Mental Hospitals and Prisons.* Boston: Beacon Press, 1984.

Costello, C. G., G. P. Belton, J. C. Abra, and B. E. Dunn. "The Amnesic and Therapeutic Effects of Bilateral and Unilateral ECT." *British Journal of Psychiatry* 116, no. 530 (1970): 69–78.

Cott, Jonathan. *On the Sea of Memory.* New York: Random House, 2005.

"Court Stays Curb on Shock Therapy." *New York Times,* January 3, 1975.

Cranford, Dr. Peter G. *But for the Grace of God: Milledgeville! The Inside Story of the World's Largest Insane Asylum.* Augusta, Ga.: Grand Pyramid Press, 1981.

Cronkite, Kathy. *On the Edge of Darkness.* New York: Delta Trade Paperbacks, 1994.

Curtis, E. "Life as Death: Hope Regained with ECT." *Psychiatric Services* 53, no. 4 (2002): 413–414.

Daniel, Walter F., and Herbert F. Crovitz. "Disorientation During Electroconvulsive Therapy: Technical, Theoretical, and Neuropsychological Issues." *Annals of the New York Academy of Science* 462 (1986): 293–306.

Daniel, Walter F., Herbert F. Crovitz, Richard D. Weiner, and Helen J. Rogers. "The Effects of ECT Modifications on Autobiographical and Verbal Memory." *Biological Psychiatry* 17, no. 8 (1982): 919–924.

Dartmouth-Hitchcock Medical Center. Electroconvulsive Therapy videotape, Department of Psychiatry.

Datto, Catherine J. "Side Effects of Electroconvulsive Therapy." *Depression and Anxiety* 12, no. 3 (2000): 130–134.

Datto, Catherine J., Stuart Levy, David S. Miller, and Ira R. Katz. "Impact of Maintenance ECT on Concentration and Memory." *Journal of ECT* 17, no. 5 (2001): 170–174.

David, H. P. "A Critique of Psychiatric and Psychological Research on Insulin Treatment in Schizophrenia." *American Journal of Psychiatry* 110, no. 10 (April 1954): 774–776.

Davis, David. "Losing the Mind: Profile of David Oaks." *Los Angeles Times Magazine,* October 26, 2003: 20–30.

"Depression: Electroconvulsive Therapy." American Academy of Family Physicians. http://familydoctor.org/058.xml.

Deutsch, Albert. *The Mentally Ill in America.* New York: Doubleday, Doran & Co., Inc., 1937.

Devanand, D. P., Linda Fitzsimons, Joan Prudic, and Harold A. Sackeim. "Subjective Side Effects During Electroconvulsive Therapy." *Convulsive Therapy* 11, no. 4 (1995): 232–240.

Devanand, D. P., and Harold A. Sackeim. "Mania as a Side-Effect of ECT." *Convulsive Therapy* 4, no. 3 (1988): 248.

Devanand, D. P., Anil K. Verma, Fughik Tirumalasetti, and Harold A. Sackeim. "Absence of Cognitive Impairment After More Than 100 Lifetime ECT Treatments." *American Journal of Psychiatry* 148, no. 7 (1991): 929–932.

de Vreede, Iris M., Huibert Burger, and Irene M. van Vliet. "Prediction of Response to ECT with Routinely Collected Data in Major Depression." *Journal of Affective Disorders* 86, nos. 2–3 (2005): 323–327.

Dew, Rachel, and W. Vaughn McCall. "Efficiency of Outpatient ECT." *Journal of ECT* 20, no. 1 (2004): 24–25.

"Dick Cavett—Actor, Author, Host: Electroconvulsive Therapy Made a Big Difference to Him." Available at: http://bipolar.about.com/cs/celebs/a/dickcavett.htm.

Dietz, Jean. "Shock Therapy's Comeback Used Against Depression: It Remains Controversial." *Boston Globe,* January 14, 1985, p. 37.

Dingxiong, He, and Li Zhuosun. "Electroconvulsive Therapy and Electric Acupuncture Convulsive Therapy in China." *Convulsive Therapy* 1, no. 4 (1985): 234–241.

D'Mello, Dale, Frederick M. Vincent, and Marvin P. Lerner. "Yawning as a Complication of Electroconvulsive Therapy and Concurrent Neuroleptic Withdrawal." *Journal of Nervous and Mental Disease* 176, no. 8 (1988): 188–189.

Donahue, Anne B. "A Basic Layperson's Guide to Decision-Making About ECT, Including Key Questions to Ask Your Doctor," undated.

———. "Electroconvulsive Therapy and Memory Loss: A Personal Journey." *Journal of ECT* 16, no. 2 (2000): 133–143.

———. Letter to Dr. Bill McMains, State of Vermont, Department of Developmental and Mental Health Services, "ECT Updates Follow-up," October 13, 2003.

Donovan, Aaron. "Learning to Live Alone and Getting to Like It." *New York Times,* December 4, 2000: B5.

Doris, Alan, Klaus Ebmeier, and Polash Shajahan. "Depressive Illness." *Lancet* 354, no. 9187 (1999): 1369–1375.

Dowd, Sheila M., Mary Jane Strong, Brian Martis, and Philip G. Janicak. "Is Repetitive Transcranial Magnetic Stimulation an Alternative to ECT for the Treatment of Depression?" *Contemporary Psychiatry* 1, no. 7 (October 2002).

Dowdy, Zachary R. "Into the Darkness Into the Light: Local Patients Report Radically Different effects from Electroshock Therapy." *Newsday,* September 16, 2001.

"Dr. Sakel Is Dead: Psychiatrist." *New York Times,* December 3, 1957, p. 35.

Duffett, Richard, Peter Hill, and Paul Lelliott. "Use of Electroconvulsive Therapy in Young People." *British Journal of Psychiatry* 175, no. 9 (1999): 228–230.

Duffett, Richard, and Paul Lelliott. "Auditing Electroconvulsive Therapy: The Third Cycle." *British Journal of Psychiatry* 172, no. 5 (1998): 401–405.

Dukakis, Kitty, with Jane Scovell. *Now You Know.* New York: Simon & Schuster, 1990.

Duke, Patty, and Gloria Hochman. *A Brilliant Madness: Living with Manic-Depressive Illness.* New York: Bantam Books, 1992.

Duraskow, D. "Interview with Dr. Max Fink." Harvard College Senior Thesis, June 30, 2003.

Durham, James. "Sources of Public Prejudice Against Electro-Convulsive Therapy." *Australian and New Zealand Journal of Psychiatry* 23, no. 4 (1989): 453–460.

Durr, Amy L., and Robert N. Golden. "Cognitive Effects of Electroconvulsive Therapy: A Clinical Review for Nurses." *Convulsive Therapy* 11, no. 3 (1995): 192–201.

Dwork, Andrew J., Victoria Arango, Mark Underwood, Boro Ilievski Gorazd Rosoklija, Harold A. Sackeim, and Sarah H. Lisanby. "Absence of Histological Lesions in Primate Models of ECT and Magnetic Seizure Therapy." *American Journal of Psychiatry* 161, no. 3 (March 2004): 576–578.

Eastwood, M. R., and J. Peacocke. "Seasonal Patterns of Suicide, Depression and Electroconvulsive Therapy." *British Journal of Psychiatry* 129 (November 1976): 472–475.

Ebaugh, Franklin G. "A Review of the Drastic Shock Therapies in the Treatment of the Psychoses." *Annals of Internal Medicine* (March 1943): 279–296.

Ebaugh, Franklin G., Clarke H. Barnacle, and Karl T. Neubuerger. "Fatalities Following Electric Convulsive Therapy: A Report of 2 Cases with Autopsy Findings." *Archives of Neurology and Psychiatry* 49, no. 107 (1943): 36–41.

Ebmeier, Klaus P., Claire Donaghey, and J. Douglas Steele. "Recent Developments and Current Controversies in Depression." *Lancet* 367 (January 14, 2006): 153–167.

"ECT in Britain: A Shameful State of Affairs." Editorial. *Lancet* (November 28, 1981): 1207–1208.

ECT statutes from across the United States.

Edelson, Edward. "ECT Elicits Controversy—and Results." *New York Daily News,* December 28, 1988.

"Editorial: The Scientific Status of Electroconvulsive Therapy." *Psychological Medicine* 9, no. 3 (August 1979): 401–408.

"Electroshock and Berkeley." *Biological Psychiatry* 18, no. 6 (1983): 609–613.

"Eliciting Users' Views of ECT in Two Mental Health Trusts with a User-Designed Questionnaire." *Journal of Mental Health* 13, no. 4 (August 2004): 403–413.

Endler, Norman S. *Holiday of Darkness: A Psychologist's Personal Journal Out of His Depression.* New York: John Wiley & Sons, 1982.

Endler, Norman S., and Emmanuel Persad. *Electroconvulsive Therapy: The Myths and the Realities.* Toronto: Hans Huber Publishers, 1988.

Enns, Murray W., and Jeffrey P. Reiss. "Electroconvulsive Therapy." *Canadian Journal of Psychiatry* 37, no. 10 (1992): 671–686.

Eranti, Savithasri V., and Declan M. McLoughlin. "Electroconvulsive Therapy—State of the Art." *British Journal of Psychiatry* 182 (January 2003): 8–9.

Evans, Rob, P. C. Naik, and S. Alikhan. "Electroconvulsive Therapy: Conflicting Advice Confuses Prescribers." *British Medical Journal* 327 (September 13, 2003): 621.

Fahy, T. J., and R. H. Latey. "Short-Term Course and Outcome of Patients Treated with Electroconvulsive Therapy: Irish and British Surveys Compared." *Convulsive Therapy* 3, no. 3 (1987): 210–217.

Farah, Andy, and W. Vaughn McCall. "Electroconvulsive Therapy Stimulus Dosing: A Survey of Contemporary Practices." *Convulsive Therapy* 9, no. 2 (1993): 90–94.

Fava, Giovanni A. "Conflict of Interest and Special Interest Groups: The Making of a Counter Culture." *Psychotherapy and Psychosomatics* 70, no. 1 (2001): 1–5.

Fayerman, Pamela. "After 130 Shock Treatments: 'They Hurt, I Don't Want It': Public Trustee's Office Investigates Riverview Case." *Vancouver Sun,* April 17, 2002, p. 1.

Fear, Christopher F., Carl S. Littlejohns, Eryl Rouse, and Paul McQuail. "Propofol Anesthesia in Electroconvulsive Therapy. Reduced Seizure Duration May Not Be Relevant." *British Journal of Psychiatry* 165, no. 4 (October 1994): 506–509.

Fear Strikes Out. Film. Directed by Robert Mulligan. Paramount Pictures, 1956.

Ferraro, Armando, and Leon Roizin. "Cerebral Morphologic Changes in Monkeys Subjected to a Large Number of Electrically Induced Convulsions (32-100)." *American Journal of Psychiatry* 106, no. 4 (1949): 278–284.

Feske, Ulrike, Benoit H. Mulsant, Paul A. Pilkonis, Paul Soloff, Diane Dolata, Harold A. Sackeim, and Roger F. Haskett. "Clinical Outcome of ECT in Patients with Major Depression and Comorbid Borderline Personality Disorder." *American Journal of Psychiatry* 161, no. 11 (2004): 2073–2080.

Field, Ellen. *The White Shirts.* M.E. Redfield Publishers, 1964.

Fink, Max. "Autobiography of L. J. Meduna." *Convulsive Therapy* 1, no. 1 (1985): 43–57 and 121–135.

———. "A Beautiful Mind and Insulin Coma: Social Constraints on Psychiatric Diagnosis and Treatment." *Harvard Review of Psychiatry* 11, no. 5 (2003): 284–290.

———. "ECT at 70: What Have We Learned?" *Psychiatric Times,* July 1, 2004.

———. "ECT in the Netherlands." *Convulsive Therapy* 11, no. 3 (1995): 224–227.

———. "ECT: Serendipity or Logical Outcome?" *Psychiatric Times* 21, no. 1 (January 2004).

———. "Effect of Anticholinergic Agent, Diethazine, on EEG and Behavior: Significance for Theory of Convulsive Therapy." *Archives of Neurology and Psychiatry* 80 (September 1958): 380–386.

———. "Efficacy and Safety of Induced Seizures (EST) in Man." *Comprehensive Psychiatry* 19, no. 1 (January/February 1978): 1–18.

———. *Electroshock: Healing Mental Illness.* New York: Oxford University Press, 1999.

———. "Electroshock Revisited." *American Scientist* 88, no. 2 (March 2000): 162.

———. "Impact of the Antipsychiatry Movement on the Revival of Electroconvulsive Therapy in the United States." *Psychiatric Clinics of North America* 14, no. 4 (1991): 793–801.

———. "Is ECT Usage Decreasing?" Editorial. *Convulsive Therapy* 3, no. 3 (1987): 171–173.

———. "Italy and Mental Illness." *New York Times,* January 4, 1989.

———. "Ladislas J. Meduna, M.D., 1896–1964." *American Journal of Psychiatry* 156, no. 11 (November 1999): 1807.

———. "A New Appreciation of ECT." *Psychiatric Times* 21, no. 4 (April 2004).

———. Overview of 20th Century Psychiatry: A Neuropsychiatrist's Perspective, 1940–2000. Course syllabus, 1999.

———. "Suicide Risk Reduced." *Psychiatric Times,* February 1, 2005.

———. "Toward a Rational Theory of Behavior." *Career Directions* 7, no. 3, Sandoz Pharmaceuticals, undated.

———. "Treating Depression." *New York Times,* October 8, 1999.

Fink, Max, and Gabrielle Carlson. "ECT and Prepubertal Children." *Journal of the American Academy of Child & Adolescent Psychiatry* 34, no. 10 (1995): 1256–1257.

Fink, Max, and Lynn Johnson. "Monitoring the Duration of Electroconvulsive Therapy Seizures." *Archives of General Psychiatry* 39, no. 10 (October 1982): 1189–1191.

Fink, Max, and Robert L. Kahn. "Behavioral Patterns in Convulsive Therapy." *Archives of General Psychiatry* 5 (1961): 30–36.

Fink, Max, Robert L. Kahn, and Martin A. Green. "Experimental Studies of the Electroshock Process." *Diseases of the Nervous System* 19, no. 3 (March 1958): 113–118.

Fisher, Seymour, Rhoda Fisher, and A. Hilkevitch. "The Conscious and Unconscious Attitudes of Psychotic Patients Towards Electric Shock Treatment." *Journal of Nervous and Mental Diseases* 118, no. 2 (August 1953): 144–152.

Foderaro, Lisa W. "With Reforms in Treatment, Shock Therapy Loses Shock." *New York Times,* July 19, 1993, sec. A, p. 1.

Folkerts, H. W., N. Michael, R. Tölle, K. Schonauer, S. Mücke, and H. Schulze-Mönking. "Electroconvulsive Therapy vs. Paroxetine in Treatment-Resistant Depression—A Randomized Study." *Acta Psychiatrica Scandinavica* 96, no. 5 (1997): 334–342.

Forbush, Bliss. *The Sheppard & Enoch Pratt Hospital, 1853–1970: A History.* Philadelphia: Lippincott Company, 1971.

Fox, Herbert A. "Continuation and Maintenance ECT." *Journal of Practical Psychiatry and Behavioral Health* (November 1996): 357–363.

———. "Electroconvulsive Therapy: An Overview." *Journal of Practical Psychiatry and Behavioral Health* (July 1996): 223–230.

———. "Extended Continuation and Maintenance ECT for Long-Lasting Episodes of Major Depression." *Journal of ECT* 17, no. 1 (March 2001): 60–64.

———. "The Natural Course of Depression: Kraepelin and Beyond." *Harvard Review of Psychiatry* 10, no. 4 (July-August 2002): 249–253.

———. "Patients' Fear of and Objection to Electroconvulsive Therapy." *Hospital and Community Psychiatry* 44, no. 4 (1993): 357–360.

Frame, Janet. *An Autobiography.* Auckland: Random Century New Zealand, 1989.

Frances. Film. Directed by Graeme Clifford. Universal, 1982.

Frank, Leonard Roy. "Electroshock: A Crime Against the Spirit." *Ethical Human Sciences and Services* 4, no. 1 (Spring 2002): 63–71.

———. "The Patient as Prisoner." In John Friedberg, *Shock Treatment Is Not Good for Your Brain.* San Francisco: Glide Publications, 1976: 54–81.

———. "The Policies and Practices of American Psychiatry Are Oppressive." *Hospital and Community Psychiatry* 37, no. 5 (1986): 497–501.

———. "Psychiatry's Unholy Trinity—Fraud, Fear, and Force: A Personal Account." *Ideas on Liberty* (November 2002): 23–27.

———. Testimony at a Public Hearing Before the Mental Health Committee of the New York State Assembly, May 18, 2001.

———, ed. *The History of Shock Treatment.* San Francisco: self-published, 1978.

Frankel, Fred H. "Current Perspectives on ECT: A Discussion." *American Journal of Psychiatry* 134, no. 9 (1977): 1014–1019.

———. "Electro-Convulsive Therapy in Massachusetts: A Task Force Report." *Massachusetts Journal of Mental Health* 3 (1973): 3–29.

Fraser, Morris. *ECT: A Clinical Guide.* New York: John Wiley & Sons, 1982.

Frederiksen, Svend-Otto, and Giacomo D'Elia. "Electroconvulsive Therapy in Sweden." *British Journal of Psychiatry* 134 (1979): 583–87.

Freeman, C.P.L. "Patients' Attitudes Toward ECT." *Psychopharmacology Bulletin* 22, no. 2 (1986): 487–490.

———. ed. *The ECT Handbook: The Second Report of the Royal College of Psychiatrists' Special Committee on ECT.* London: Royal College of Psychiatrists, 1995.

Freeman, C.P.L., J. V. Basson, and A. Crighton. "Double-Blind Controlled Trial of Electroconvulsive Therapy (ECT) and Simulated ECT in Depressive Illness." *Lancet* 1, no. 8067 (1978): 738–740.

Freeman, C.P.L., and R. E. Kendell. "ECT: I: Patients' Experiences and Attitudes." *British Journal of Psychiatry* 137 (July 1980): 8–16.

Freeman, C.P.L., D. Weeks, and R. E. Kendell. "ECT: II: Patients Who Complain." *British Journal of Psychiatry* 137 (July 1980): 17–25.

Freeman, Lucy. "Advantages Noted on Shock Therapy." *New York Times*, December 18, 1949, p. 63.

———. "Shock Treatment Held Not Enough." *New York Times*, April 14, 1949.

Friedberg, John. "Electroshock Therapy: Let's Stop Blasting the Brain." *Psychology Today*, August 1975.

———. "Shock Treatment, Brain Damage, and Memory Loss: A Neurological Perspective." *American Journal of Psychiatry* 134, no. 9 (September 1977): 1010–1014.

———. *Shock Treatment Is Not Good for Your Brain*. San Francisco: Glide Publications, 1976.

Funk, Wendy. *What Difference Does it Make? (The Journey of a Soul Survivor)*. Whitehorse, Yukon: Wild Flower Publishing, 1998.

Gabbard, Glen O., and Krin Gabbard. *Psychiatry and the Cinema*. Washington, D.C.: American Psychiatric Press Inc., 1999.

Gagne Jr., Gerard G., Martin J. Furman, Linda L. Carpenter, and Lawrence H. Price. "Efficacy of Continuation ECT and Antidepressant Drugs Compared to Long-Term Antidepressants Alone in Depressed Patients." *American Journal of Psychiatry* 157, no. 12 (December 2000): 1960–1965.

"Gains Made in Help to Schizophrenics." *New York Times*, May 11, 1949, p. 8.

Gangadhar, B. N., N. Janakiramaiah, D. K. Subbakrishna, J. Praveen, and Ashok K. Reddy. "Twice Versus Thrice Weekly ECT in Melancholia: A Double-Blind Prospective Comparison." *Journal of Affective Disorders* 27, no. 4 (1993): 273–278.

Gass, John P. "The Knowledge and Attitudes of Mental Health Nurses to Electro-Convulsive Therapy." *Journal of Advanced Nursing* 27, no. 1 (1998): 83–90.

Gazdag, G., N. Kocsis, and A. Lipcsey. "Rates of Electroconvulsive Therapy Use in Hungary in 2002." *Journal of ECT* 20, no. 1 (2004): 42–44.

Ghaziuddin, Neera, Cheryl A. King, Michael W. Naylor, Mohammed Ghaziuddin, Nadira Chaudhary, Bruno Giordani, John R. Dequardo, Rajiv Tandon, and John Greden. "Electroconvulsive Treatment in Adolescents with Pharmacotherapy-Refractory Depression." *Journal of Child and Adolescent Psychopharmacology* 6, no. 4 (1996): 259–271.

Ghaziuddin, Neera, Stanley P. Kutcher, Penelope Knapp, William Bernet, Valerie Arnold, Joseph Beitchman, R. Scott Benson, Oscar Bukstein, Joan Kinlan, Jon McClellan, David Rue, Jon A. Shaw, and Saundra Stock. "Practice Parameter for

Use of Electroconvulsive Therapy with Adolescents (AACAP Official Action)." *Journal of the American Academy of Child & Adolescent Psychiatry* 43, no. 12 (December 1, 2004): 1521–1539.

Ghaziuddin, Neera, Donna Laughrin, and Bruno Giodani. "Cognitive Side Effects in Electroconvulsive Therapy in Adolescents." *Journal of Child and Adolescent Psychopharmacology* 10, no. 4 (2000): 269–276.

Glass, Richard M. "Electroconvulsive Therapy: Time to Bring It Out of the Shadows." *Journal of the American Medical Association* 285, no. 10 (2001): 1346–1348.

Glen, Tom, and Allan I. F. Scott. "Rates of Electroconvulsive Therapy Use in Edinburgh (1992–1997)." *Journal of Affective Disorders* 54, nos. 1–2 (1999): 81–85.

———. "Variation in Rates of Electroconvulsive Therapy Use Among Consultant Teams in Edinburgh (1993–1996)." *Journal of Affective Disorders* 58, no. 1 (2000): 75–78.

Glueck Jr., Bernard C., Harry Reiss, and Louis E. Bernard. "Regressive Electric Shock Therapy: Preliminary Report on 100 Cases." *Psychiatric Quarterly* 31, no. 1 (January 1957): 117–136.

Goldberg, Carey. "Early McLean Tests Show Brain Scan Eases Depression," *Boston Globe,* January 1, 2004.

Goldman, Douglas. "Brief Stimulus Electric Shock Therapy." *Journal of Nervous and Mental Disorders* 110 (1949): 36–45.

Goleman, Daniel. "A Panel Backs Punishment Therapy." *New York Times,* September 14, 1989.

———. "The Quiet Comeback of Electroshock Therapy." *New York Times,* August 2, 1990.

Goodman, Wayne K., Matthew V. Rudorfer, and Jack D. Maser. *Obsessive-Compulsive Disorder: Contemporary Issues in Treatment.* Mahwah, N.J.: Lawrence Erlbaum Associates, 2000.

Gordon, Hirsch L. "Fifty Shock Therapy Theories." *Military Surgeon* 103 (1948): 397–401.

Government Statistical Service, Department of Health (UK). *Electro Convulsive Therapy: Survey Covering the Period from January 1999 to March 1999.* London: Department of Health, September 1999.

———. *Electro Convulsive Therapy: Survey Covering the Period from January 2002 to March 2002.* London: Department of Health, August 2002.

Graham, Tom. "Shock Therapy: Positive and Negative Changes." *Washington Post,* June 6, 2000, sec. Z, p. 16.

Grahn, Allen R. "Summary of Presentation to FDA Neurology Panel, Study of Electroconvulsive Therapy Device Safety and Efficacy." Utah Biomedical Test Laboratory, October 15, 1976.

Gralnick, Alexander. "Fatalities Associated with Electric Shock Treatment of Psychoses: Report of Two Cases with Autopsy Observations in One of Them." *Archives of Neurology and Psychiatry* 51 (1944): 397–402.

Gray, Francine du Plessix. "Prophets of Seduction." *The New Yorker,* November 4, 1996.

Greenberg, Robert M., and Charles H. Kellner. "Electroconvulsive Therapy: A Selected Review." *American Journal of Geriatric Psychiatry* 13, no. 4 (2005): 268–281.

Greenhalgh, Joanne, Chris Knight, D. Hind, C. Beverly, and Stephen Walters. "Clinical and Cost-Effectiveness of Electroconvulsive Therapy for Depressive Illness, Schizophrenia, Catatonia and Mania: Systematic Reviews and Economic Modeling Studies," *Health Technology Assessment* 9, no. 9 (March 2005): 1–156.

Greenhalgh, Joanne, Chris Knight, D. Hind, C. Beverly, and Stephen Walters. *Electroconvulsive Therapy (ECT) for Depressive Illness, Schizophrenia, Catatonia and Mania.* Sheffield, UK: Trent Institute for Health Services, 2002.

Gregory, S., C. R. Shawcross, and D. Gill. "The Nottingham ECT Study: A Double-Blind Comparison of Bilateral, Unilateral and Simulated ECT in Depressive Illness." *British Journal of Psychiatry* 146 (1985): 520–524.

Grob, Gerald N. *The Mad Among Us: A History of the Care of America's Mentally Ill.* New York: The Free Press, 1994.

Grobe, Jeanine, ed. *Beyond Bedlam: Contemporary Women Psychiatric Survivors Speak Out.* Chicago: Third Side Press, 1995.

Grosser, George H., Doris T. Pearsall, Cindy L. Fisher, and Lois Geremonte. "The Regulation of Electroconvulsive Therapy in Massachusetts: A Follow-up." *Massachusetts Journal of Mental Health* 5 (1975): 12–25.

Group for the Advancement of Psychiatry. "Revised Electro-Shock Therapy Report." Report No. 15, August 1950, New York.

———. "Shock Therapy." Report No. 1, September 15, 1947, New York.

Grunhaus, L., O. Dolberg, and M. Lustig. "Relapse and Recurrence Following a Course of ECT: Reasons for Concern and Strategies for Further Investigation." *Journal of Psychiatric Research* 29, no. 3 (1995): 165–172.

Grunhaus, Leon, Pinhas N. Dannon, Shaul Schreiber, Ornah H. Dolberg, Revital Amiaz, Reuven Ziv, and Eli Lefkifker. "Repetitive Transcranial Magnetic Stimulation Is as Effective as Electroconvulsive Therapy in the Treatment of Nondelusional Major Depressive Disorder: An Open Study." *Biological Psychiatry* 47, no. 4 (2000): 314–324.

Guttmacher, Laurence B. *Psychopharmacology & Electroconvulsive Therapy.* Washington, D.C.: American Psychiatric Press, Inc., 1994.

Halliday, Graeme, and Gordon Johnson. "Training to Administer Electroconvulsive Therapy: A Survey of Attitudes and Experiences." *Australian and New Zealand Journal of Psychiatry* 29, no. 1 (1995): 133–138.

Hamilton, Max. "A Rating Scale for Depression." *Journal of Neurology, Neurosurgery and Psychiatry* 23, no. 1 (February 1960): 56–62.

Harkavy, Ward. "Watts Up: More New Yorkers Getting Zapped by Court-Ordered Electroshock." *Village Voice*, May 16, 2001.

Harms, Ernest. "The Origin and Early History of Electrotherapy and Electroshock." *American Journal of Psychiatry* 111, no. 12 (June 1955): 933–934.

Harrison, Emma. "Shock Treatment 'Ugly' to Pioneer." *New York Times*, April 24, 1959, p. 25.

The Hemingway Resource Center, http://www.lostgeneration.com.

Hermann, Richard C. "Variation in Psychiatric Practices: Implications for Health Care Policy and Financing." *Harvard Review of Psychiatry* 4, no. 2 (1996): 98–101.

Hermann, Richard C., Robert A. Dorwart, Claudia W Hoover, and Jeremy Brody. "Variation in ECT Use in the United States." *American Journal of Psychiatry* 152, no. 6 (June 1995): 869–875.

Hermann, Richard C., Susan L. Ettner, Robert A. Dorwart, Claudia W. Hoover, and Elaine Yeung. "Characteristics of Psychiatrists Who Perform ECT." *American Journal of Psychiatry* 155, no. 7 (1998): 889–894.

Hermann, Richard C., Susan L. Ettner, Robert A. Dorwart, Nancy Langman-Dorwart, and Stephen Kleinman. "Diagnoses of Patients Treated with ECT: A Comparison of Evidence-Based Standards with Reported Use." *Psychiatric Services* 50, no. 8 (1999): 1059–1065.

Heshe, J., and E. Roeder. "Electroconvulsive Therapy in Denmark." *British Journal of Psychiatry* 128 (1976): 241–245.

Hickie, I., C. Mason, G. Parker, and H. Brodaty. "Prediction of ECT Response: Validation of a Refined Sign-Based (CORE) System for Defining Melancholia." *British Journal of Psychiatry* 169, no. 1 (1996): 68–74.

Hill, Gladwin. "Ideas and Trends: Now, Therapy by the Ballot." *New York Times*, October 31, 1982.

Himwich, Harold E. "Electroshock: A Round Table Discussion." *American Journal of Psychiatry* 100 (1943): 361–364.

Hochmann, Anndee. "The Return of Shock Therapy." *Health* (January/February 2004): 96–98.

Hoffenberg, Noah. "Electroconvulsive Therapy: It's Not Voodoo Science." Available online at: http://www.healthquarterly.com/Summer_2004/default.asp?id=article04.

"Hospital Cites Aid for Mental Cases." *New York Times*, June 11, 1948, p. 20.

Hotchner, A. E. *Papa Hemingway: A Personal Memoir.* New York: Random House, 1955.

Hubbard, L. Ron. *Dianetics: The Modern Science of Mental Health*. Los Angeles: Bridge Publications, Inc., 1950.

Huston, Paul E., and Lillian M. Lochere. "Manic-Depressive Psychosis: Course When Treated and Untreated with Electric Shock." *Archives of Neurology and Psychiatry* 60 (1948): 37–48.

Ikeji, O. C., J. U. Ohaeri, R. O. Osahon, and R. O. Agidee. "Naturalistic Comparative Study of Outcome and Cognitive Effects of Unmodified Electro-Convulsive Therapy in Schizophrenia, Mania and Severe Depression in Nigeria." *East African Medical Journal* 76, no. 11 (1999): 644–650.

Illinois Department of Human Services, "Summary of Annual Reports Compiled by DHS on ECT," 1998–2003.

Impastato, David J. "Prevention of Fatalities in Electroshock Therapy." *Diseases of the Nervous System* 18, no. 2 (1957): 34–74.

———. "The Story of the First Electroshock Treatment." *American Journal of Psychiatry* 116 (1960): 1113–1114.

Impastato, David J., and Renato Almansi. "The Electrofit in the Treatment of Mental Disease." *Journal of Nervous and Mental Diseases* 96 (October 1942): 395–408.

Infinite Mind, The. Public radio show, "Electroconvulsive Therapy," no. 373, Week of May 5, 2005.

Institute of Psychiatry. "Reviews of Consumers' Perspectives on Electro Convulsive Therapy," Service User Research Enterprise, Department of Health, Great Britain, Final Report, January 2002.

"Into the Light." *People*, March 28, 2005.

Iodice, Aline J., Aaron G. Dunn, Peter Rosenquist, Doreen L. Hughes, and W. Vaughn McCall. "Stability over Time of Patients' Attitudes Toward ECT." *Psychiatry Research* 117, no. 1 (2003): 89–91.

Ishimoto, Yasuhito, Akira Imakura, and Hiroshi Nakayama. "Practice of Electroconvulsive Therapy at University Hospital, the University of Tokushima School of Medicine from 1975 to 1997." *Journal of Medical Investigation* 47, nos. 3–4 (August 2000): 123–127.

Isometsa, Erkki T., Markus M. Henriksson, Martti E. Heikkinen, and Jouko K. Lonnqvist. "Completed Suicide and Recent Electroconvulsive Therapy in Finland." *Convulsive Therapy* 12, no. 3 (1996): 152–155.

Jackson, Joyce. "Electroconvulsive Therapy: Problems and Prejudices." *Convulsive Therapy* 11, no. 3 (1995): 179–181.

Jamison, Kay Redfield. *An Unquiet Mind: A Memoir of Moods and Madness*. New York: Vintage Books, 1995.

———. *Touched with Fire: Manic-Depressive Illness and the Artistic Temperament.* New York: Free Press Paperbacks, 1993.

Janakiramaiah, N., B. N. Gangadhar, P. J. Naga Venkatesha Murthy, M. G. Harish, D. K. Subbakrishna, and A. Vedamurthachar. "Antidepressant Efficacy of Sudarshan Kriya Yoga (SKY) in Melancholia: A Randomized Comparison with Electroconvulsive Therapy (ECT) and Imipramine." *Journal of Affective Disorders* 57, nos. 1–3 (January–March 2000): 255–259.

Janakiramaiah, N., S. Motreja, B. N. Gangadhar, D. K. Subbakrishna, and G. Parameshwara. "Once vs. Three Times Weekly ECT in Melancholia: A Randomized Controlled Trial." *Acta Psychiatrica Scandinavica* 98, no. 4 (1998): 316–320.

Janicak, Philip G., John M. Davis, Robert D. Gibbons, Stephen Ericksen, Sidney Chang, and Peter Gallagher. "Efficacy of ECT: A Meta-Analysis." *American Journal of Psychiatry* 142, no. 3 (1985): 297–302.

Janicak, Philip G., Sheila M. Dowd, Brian Martis, Danesh Alam, Dennis Beedle, Jack Krasuski, Mary Jane Strong, Rajiv Sharma, Cherise Rosen, and Marlos Viana. "Repetitive Transcranial Magnetic Stimulation Versus Electroconvulsive Therapy for Major Depression: Preliminary Results of a Randomized Trial." *Society of Biological Psychiatry* 51 (April 15, 2002): 659–667.

Janis, Irving L. "Memory Loss Following Electric Convulsive Treatments." *Journal of Personality* 17 (1948): 29–32.

———. "Psychological Effects of Electric Convulsive Treatments, (I. Post-Treatment Amnesias)." *Journal of Nervous and Mental Disease* 3, no. 5 (May 1950): 359–382.

Jessner, Lucie, and V. Gerard Ryan. *Shock Treatment in Psychiatry: A Manual.* New York: Grune & Stratton, 1941.

Johnstone, Lucy. "Adverse Psychological Effects of ECT." *Journal of Mental Health* 8, no. 1 (1999): 69–85.

"Jury Rules on Death: Father of Slain Chicago Boys Died During Shock Therapy." *New York Times,* November 13, 1955.

Kalinowsky, Lothar B. "The Discoveries of Somatic Treatments in Psychiatry: Facts and Myths." *Comprehensive Psychiatry* 21, no. 6 (November/December 1980): 428–434.

———. "Organic Psychotic Syndromes Occurring During Electric Convulsive Therapy." *Archives of Neurology and Psychiatry* 53 (1945): 269–273.

Kalinowsky, Lothar B., Hanns Hippius, and Helmfried E. Klein. *Biological Treatments in Psychiatry.* New York: Grune & Stratton, 1982.

Kalinowsky, Lothar B., and Paul H. Hoch. *Shock Treatments and Other Somatic Procedures in Psychiatry.* New York: Grune & Stratton, 1950.

Katona, C.L.E., and C. R. Aldridge. "Prediction of ECT Response." *Neuropharmacology* 23, no. 2B (1984): 281–283.

Katzenelbogen, Solomon. "Critical Appraisal of the 'Shock Therapies' in the Major Psychoses and Psychoneuroses, III—Convulsive Therapy." *Psychiatry* 3 (1940): 409–420.

Kellner, Charles H. "ECT at Mid-Decade: Two Steps Forward, One Step Back." *Convulsive Therapy* 11, no. 1 (1995): 1–2.

———. "Left Unilateral ECT: Still a Viable Option?" *Convulsive Therapy* 13, no. 2 (1997): 65–67.

———. "Towards the Modal ECT Treatment." *Journal of ECT* 17 no. 1 (2001): 1–2.

Kellner, Charles H., Max Fink, Rebecca Knapp, Georgio Petrides, Mustafa Husain, Teresa Rummans, Martina Mueller, Hilary Bernstein, Keith Rasmussen, Kevin O'Connor, Glenn Smith, A. John Rush, Melanie Biggs, Shawn McClintock, Samuel Bailine, and Chitra Malur. "Relief of Expressed Suicidal Intent by ECT: A Consortium for Research in ECT Study." *American Journal of Psychiatry* 162, no. 5 (2005): 977–982.

Kennedy, Cyril J. C., and David Anchel. "Regressive Electric-Shock in Schizophrenics Refractory to Other Shock Therapies." *Psychiatric Quarterly* 22, no. 1 (1948): 317–320.

Kesey, Ken. *One Flew Over the Cuckoo's Nest*. New York: Viking Press, 1962.

Khanna, Suman, B. N. Gangadhar, Vinod Sinha, P. N. Rajendra, and S. M. Channabasavanna. "Electroconvulsive Therapy in Obsessive-Compulsive Disorder." *Convulsive Therapy* 4, no. 4 (1988): 314–320.

Kirkwood, Julie. "To Remember, or Forget? Motivation Varied among Authors Recounting Horror of Danvers State Hospital." *Lawrence* (Massachusetts) *Eagle-Tribune,* June 28, 2005.

Klerman, Gerald L. "The Psychiatric Patient's Right to Effective Treatment: Implications of Osheroff v. Chestnut Lodge." *American Journal of Psychiatry* 147, no. 4 (1990): 409–418.

Kobayashi, Masahito, and Alvaro Pascual-Leone. "Transcranial Magnetic Stimulation in Neurology." *Lancet* 2 (March 2003): 145–156.

Kramer, Barry Alan. "Use of ECT in California, Revisited: 1984–1994." *Journal of ECT* 15, no. 4 (December 1999): 245–251.

Kroessler, David, and Barry S. Fogel. "Electroconvulsive Therapy for Major Depression in the Oldest Old: Effects of Medical Comorbidity on Post-Treatment Survival." *American Journal of Geriatric Psychiatry* 1, no. 1 (1993): 30–37.

Krueger, Richard B., Harold A. Sackeim, and Elkan R. Gamzu. "Pharmacological Treatment of the Cognitive Side Effects of ECT: A Review." *Psychopharmacology Bulletin* 28, no. 4 (1992): 409–424.

Krystal, Andrew D., Mike West, Raquel Prado, Henry Greenside, Scott Zoldi, and

Richard D. Weiner. "EEG Effects of ECT: Implications for rTMS." *Depression and Anxiety* 12, no. 3 (2000): 157–165.

Kujala, Ilkka, Berit Rosenvinge, and Svein Ivar Bekkelund. "Clinical Outcome and Adverse Effects of Electroconvulsive Therapy in Elderly Psychiatric Patients." *Journal of Geriatric Psychiatry and Neurology* 15, no. 2 (Summer 2002): 73–76.

Lam v. Upjohn Co. 1995 U.S. Dist. LEXIS 7642, April 21, 1995.

Lambourn, J., and D. Gill. "A Controlled Comparison of Simulated and Real ECT." *British Journal of Psychiatry* 133 (1978): 514–519.

Langsley, Donald G., and Joel Yager. "The Definition of a Psychiatrist: Eight Years Later." *American Journal of Psychiatry* 145, no. 4 (April 1988): 469–475.

Latey, R. H., and T. J. Fahy. "Electroconvulsive Therapy in the Republic of Ireland 1982: A Summary of Findings." *British Journal of Psychiatry* 147 (October 1985): 438–439.

Lauber, Christopher, Carlos Nordt, Luis Falcato, and Wulf Rossler. "Can a Seizure Help? The Public's Attitude Toward Electroconvulsive Therapy." *Psychiatric Research* 134, no. 2 (2005): 205–209.

Lauter, H., and H. Sauer. "Electroconvulsive Therapy: A German Perspective." *Convulsive Therapy* 3, no. 3 (1987): 204–209.

Lawrence, Juli. *Voices from Within: A Study of ECT and Patient Perceptions.* Available at www.ect.org.

"Lawyer Recounts Peronist Torture." *New York Times,* August 18, 1949, p. 9.

Lebensohn, Zigmond M. "Electroconvulsive Therapy: Psychiatry's Villain or Hero?" *American Journal of Social Psychiatry* 4, no. 4 (Fall 1984): 39–43.

———. "The History of Electroconvulsive Therapy in the United States and Its Place in American Psychiatry: A Personal Memoir." *Comprehensive Psychiatry* 40, no. 3 (1999): 173–181.

———. "Letter to Editor in Response to Elizabeth Wertz." *Washington Post,* March 4, 1973.

———. "Problems in Obtaining Informed Consent for Electroshock Therapy." In *Readings in Law and Psychiatry.* Edited by Richard C. Allen. Baltimore: Johns Hopkins University Press, 1975.

Lehmann, H. E. "Therapeutic Results with Chlorpromazine (Largactil) in Psychiatric Conditions." *Canadian Medication Association Journal* 72 (January 15, 1955): 91–99.

Lerer, Bernard, Baruch Shapira, Avraham Calev, Hurith Tubi, Heinz Drexler, Seth Kindler, David Lidsky, and Joseph E. Schwartz. "Antidepressant and Cognitive Effects of Twice- Versus Three-Time-Weekly ECT." *American Journal of Psychiatry* 152, no. 4 (1995): 564–570.

Letemendia, F. J., N. J. Delva, M. Rodenburg, J. S. Lawson, J. Inglis, J. J. Waldron, and

D. W. Lywood. "Therapeutic Advantage of Bifrontal Electrode Placement in ECT." *Psychological Medicine* 23, no. 2 (1993): 349–360.

Levant, Oscar. *The Memoirs of an Amnesiac.* New York: G. P. Putnam's Sons, 1965.

Levenson, James L., and Allan Brock Willett. "Milieu Reactions to ECT." *Psychiatry* 45, no. 4 (November 1982): 298–306.

Levin, Martin. "A Reader's Report." *New York Times,* February 4, 1962, p. 214.

Lewis, Nolan D. C. "The Present Status of Shock Therapy of Mental Disorders." *Bulletin of the New York Academy of Medicine* (April 1943): 227–243.

Li, Xingbao, Ziad Nahas, Berry Anderson, F. Andrew Kozel, and Mark S. George. "Can Left Prefrontal rTMS Be Used as a Maintenance Treatment for Depression?" *Depression and Anxiety* 20, no. 2 (2004): 98–100.

"Life in the Loony Bin," *Time,* February 16, 1962.

Linington, Alison, and Brian Harris. "Fifty Years of Electroconvulsive Therapy." *British Medical Journal* 297 (November 26, 1988): 1354–1355.

Lippman, Steven, Manoochehr Manshadi, Mark Wehry, Ryland Byrd, Wally Past, William Keller, James Schuster, Sandra Elam, David Meyer, and Regina O' Daniel.. "1,250 Electroconvulsive Treatments Without Evidence of Brain Injury." *British Journal of Psychiatry* 147 (1985): 203–204.

Lisanby, Sarah H., ed. *Brain Stimulation in Psychiatric Treatment.* Washington, D.C.: American Psychiatric Publishing, Inc., 2004.

———. "Implications for the Neural Circuitry of Depression." *Psychological Medicine* 33, no. 1 (January 2003): 7–13.

———. "Update on Magnetic Seizure Therapy: A Novel Form of Convulsive Therapy." *Journal of ECT* 18, no. 4 (December 2002): 182–188.

Lisanby, Sarah H., Catherine F. Datto, and Martin P. Szuba. "ECT and TMS: Past, Present, and Future." *Depression and Anxiety* 12, no. 3 (2000): 115–117.

Lisanby, Sarah H., D. P. Devanand, Mitchell S. Nobler, Joan Prudic, Linda Mullen, and Harold A. Sackeim. "Exceptionally High Seizure Threshold: ECT Device Limitations." *Convulsive Therapy* 12, no. 3 (1996): 156–164.

Lisanby, Sarah H., Bruce Luber, Tarique Perera, and Harold A. Sackeim. "Transcranial Magnetic Stimulation: Applications in Basic Neuroscience and Neuropsychopharmacology." *International Journal of Neuropsychopharmacology* 3, no. 3 (September 2000): 259–273.

Lisanby, Sarah H., Bruce Luber, Harold A. Sackeim, A. D. Finck, and Charles Schroeder. "Deliberate Seizure Induction with Repetitive Transcranial Magnetic Stimulation in Nonhuman Primates." *Archives of General Psychiatry* 58, no. 2 (February 1991): 199–200.

Lisanby, Sarah H., Bruce Luber, Thomas E. Schlaepfer, and Harold Sackeim. "Safety and Feasibility of Magnetic Seizure Therapy (MST) in Major Depression: Randomized Within-Subject Comparison with Electroconvulsive Therapy." *Neuropsychopharmacology* 28, no. 10 (October 2003): 1852–1865.

Lisanby, Sarah H., Jill H. Maddox, Joan Prudic, D. P. Devanand, and Harold A. Sackeim. "The Effects of Electroconvulsive Therapy on Memory of Autobiographical and Public Events." *Archives of General Psychiatry* 57, no. 6 (June 2000): 581–590.

Lisanby, Sarah H., and O. G. Morales. "Invited Review of Electroconvulsive Therapy by Richard Abrams." *Psychological Medicine* 33 (2003):1485–1487.

Lisanby, Sarah H., T. Moscrip, O. G. Morales, B. Luber, C. Schroeder, and H. A. Sackeim. "Neurophysiological Characterization of MST in Non-Human Primates." *Supplements to Clinical Neurophysiology* 56 (2003): 81–99.

Lisanby, Sarah H., and Harold A. Sackeim. "New Developments in Convulsive Therapy for Major Depression." *Epilepsy & Behavior* 2, no. 3 (June 2001): S68–S73.

Lisanby, Sarah H., Thomas E. Schlaepfer, Hans-Ulrich Fisch, and Harold A. Sackeim. "Magnetic Seizure Therapy of Major Depression." Letters to Editor. *Archives of General Psychiatry* 58, no. 3 (March 2001): 303–304.

Liston, E. H., B. H. Guze, L. R. Baxter, S. T. Richeimer, and M. H. Gold. "Motor Versus EEG Seizure Duration in ECT." *Biological Psychiatry* 24, no. 1 (May 1988): 94–96.

Little, John D. "ECT in the Asia Pacific Region: What Do We Know?" *Journal of ECT,* 19, no. 2 (June 2003): 93–97.

Lonsdale, Sarah. "ECT Shocks to the Health System; Is Electroshock Therapy a Real Lifesaver or a Mind Thief?" *The Independent,* June 16, 1998: Features, p. 14.

Lowinger, Louis, and James H. Huddleson. "Complications in Electric Shock Therapy." *American Journal of Psychiatry* 102 (March 1946): 594–598.

Lydon, Christopher. "Eagleton Tells of Shock Therapy on Two Occasions." *New York Times,* July 26, 1972, p. 1.

Mahler, Susan. "Shock Therapy." *Threepenny Review* 90 (Summer 2002): 4–7.

"Making Sense of ECT." National Association of Mental Health. http://www.mind.org.uk/Information/Booklets/Making sense/ECT.htm.

Malsch, Evamarie, Laura Ho, Michael J. Booth, and Elain Allen. "Survey of Anesthetic Coverage of Electroconvulsive Therapy in the State of Pennsylvania." *Convulsive Therapy* 7, no. 4 (1991): 262–274.

Mann, Stephen C., Stanley N. Caroff, Henry R. Bleier, Eduardo Antelo, and Hyong Un. "Electroconvulsive Therapy of the Lethal Catatonia Syndrome." *Convulsive Therapy* 6, no. 3 (1990): 239–247.

Manning, Martha. "Intimacy and Stuff: Psychotherapists Agree That It's Not Particularly Easy." *New York Times,* November 2, 1997: A1.

———. *Undercurrents: A Life Beneath the Surface.* New York: HarperCollins, 1994.

Markowitz, John C. "Shock Therapy." *New York Times,* December 20, 1987.

Martis, Brian, Danesh Alam, Sheila M. Down, S. Kristin Hill, Rajiv P. Sharma, Cherise Rosen, Neil Pliskin, Eileen Martin, Valerie Carson, and Philip G. Janicak. "Neurocognitive Effects of Repetitive Transcranial Magnetic Stimulation in Severe Major Depression." *Clinical Neurophysiology* 114, no. 6 (June 2003): 1125–1132.

Mayberg, Helen S., Andres M. Lozano, Valerie Voon, Heather E. McNeely, David Seminowicz, Clement Hamani, Jason M. Schwalb, and Sidney H. Kennedy. "Deep Brain Stimulation for Treatment-Resistant Depression." *Neuron* 45, no. 5 (2005): 651–660.

Mayo Foundation for Medical Education and Research. "Electroconvulsive Therapy: Dramatic Relief for Severe Mental Illness." July 16, 2004. Available at http://www.mayoclinic.com.

Mayur, P. M., B. N. Gangadhar, N. Janakiramaiah, and D. K. Subbakrishna. "Motor Seizure Monitoring During ECT." *British Journal of Psychiatry* 174, no. 3 (March 1999): 270–272.

McCall, W. Vaughn. "Concerns over Antidepressant Medications and Suicide: What Does It Mean for ECT?" *Journal of ECT* 21, no. 1 (2005): 1–2.

——. "Physical Treatments in Psychiatry: Current and Historical Use in the Southern United States." *Southern Medical Journal* 82, no. 3 (March 1989): 345–351.

McCall, W. Vaughn, Aaron G. Dunn, and Charles H. Kellner. "Recent Advances in the Science of ECT: Can the Findings Be Generalized?" *Journal of ECT* 16, no. 4 (2000): 323–326.

McCall, W. Vaughn, Aaron Dunn, Peter B. Rosenquist, and Doreen Hughes. "Markedly Suprathreshold Right Unilateral ECT versus Minimally Suprathreshold Bilateral ECT: Antidepressant and Memory Effects." *Journal of ECT* 18, no. 3 (2002): 126–129.

McCall, W. Vaughn, Joan Prudic, Mark Olfson, and Harold Sackeim. "Health-Related Quality of Life Following ECT in a Large Community Sample." *Journal of Affective Disorders* 90 (2006): 269–274.

McCall, W. Vaughn, David M. Reboussin, Richard D. Weiner, and Harold A. Sackeim. "Titrated Moderately Suprathreshold vs Fixed High-Dose Right Unilateral Electroconvulsive Therapy: Acute Antidepressant and Cognitive Effects." *Archives of General Psychiatry* 57, no. 5 (May 2000): 438–444.

McDonald, Breanna C. "Attached Confidential Neuropsychological Evaluation." Dartmouth Medical School, Department of Psychiatry, March 24, 2003.

McDonald, William M., and Benjamin Greenberg. "Electroconvulsive Therapy in the Treatment of Neuropsychiatric Conditions and Transcranial Magnetic Stimulation as a Pathophysiological Probe in Neuropsychiatry." *Depression and Anxiety* 12, no. 3 (2000): 135–143.

McDougle, C. J., and K. H. Walsh. "Treatment of Refractory OCD." In Naomi

Fineberg, ed., *Obsessive Compulsive Disorder: A Practical Guide.* London: Martin Dunitz, 2001.

McElhiney, Martin C., Bobba J. Moody, Barbara L. Steif, Joan Prudic, D. P. Devanand, Mitchell S. Nobler, and Harold A. Sackeim. "Autobiographical Memory and Mood: Effects of Electroconvulsive Therapy." *Neuropsychology* 9, no. 4 (1995): 501–517.

McLean Hospital Archives. "Electric Shock Treatment Procedure." Undated. Belmont, Massachusetts.

———. "General Preparatory Requirements and Considerations for Electric Shock Therapy at the McLean Hospital." Undated.

———. Letter from Dr. Stanley Cobb to Dr. William Franklin Wood at McLean, July 8, 1941.

———. Letter to Dr. K. J. Tillotson from Victor Guillemin, January 28, 1941.

———. Letter from W. Franklin Wood, M.D./Director, to U.S. surgeon general, March 14, 1942, transmitting report on shock therapies.

Mecta Corporation. "Ultrabrief ECT—Ensuring Efficacy While Markedly Reducing Cognitive Side Effects."

Meduna, L. J. "Autobiography of L. J. Meduna: Part Two." *Convulsive Therapy* 1, no. 2 (1985): 121–135.

Meduna, Laszlo Joseph. "The Convulsive Treatment: A Reappraisal," in Arthur M. Sacklen's *The Great Physiodynamic Therapies in Psychiatry: An Historic Reappraisal,* pp. 76–90. New York: Hoeber, 1956.

Mental Disability Rights International & Asociación por Derechos Humano. "Human Rights and Mental Health in Peru." September 2004, Lima, Peru. Available online at http://www.mdri.org/pdf/Peru%20Report%20-%20Eng%20-%20Final.pdf.

Mental Health Organizations. Official position papers on ECT—and clarifying e-mails from spokespeople—from the Depression and Bipolar Support Alliance, National Mental Health Association, and National Alliance for the Mentally Ill.

"Mental Ills Aided by Shock Therapy." *New York Times,* June 3, 1948, p. 20.

Meyers, Jeffrey. *Hemingway: A Biography.* New York: Da Capa Press, 1999.

Michel, Ernest W. "I Saw Him in Action." In *The Nazi Doctors.* ed. Robert Jay Lifton New York: Basic Books, 1986.

Miller, Alexander L., Raymond A. Faber, John P. Hatch, and Harold E. Alexander. "Factors Affecting Amnesia, Seizure Durations and Efficacy in ECT." *American Journal of Psychiatry* 142, no. 6 (1985): 692–696.

Miller, Laura J. "Use of Electroconvulsive Therapy During Pregnancy." *Hospital and Community Psychiatry* 45, no. 5 (1994): 444–450.

Millet, John A. P., and Eric P. Mosse. "On Certain Psychological Aspects of Electroshock Therapy." *Psychosomatic Medicine* 6 (1944): 226–236.

Mills, Mark J., Doris T. Pearsall, Jerome A. Yesavage, and Carl Salzman. "Electroconvulsive Therapy in Massachusetts." *American Journal of Psychiatry* 141, no. 4 (1984): 534–538.

Milstein, Victor, and Iver F. Small. "Electroconvulsive Therapy: Attitudes and Experience—A Survey of Indiana Psychiatrists." *Convulsive Therapy* 1, no. 2 (1985): 89–100.

Mogilner, A. Y., and A. R. Rezai. "Brain Stimulation: History, Current Clinical Application, and Future Prospects." *Acta Neurochirurgica* (2003): 115–120.

Moise, Frantz N., and Georgios Petrides. "Case Study: Electroconvulsive Therapy in Adolescents." *Journal of the American Academy of Child & Adolescent Psychiatry* 35, no. 3 (March 1996): 312–317.

Moser, D. J., R. E. Jorge, F. Manes, S. Paradiso, M. L. Benjamin, and R. G. Robinson. "Improved Executive Function Following Repetitive Transcranial Magnetic Stimulation." *Neurology* 58, no. 8 (2002): 1288–1290.

Mosher, Loren R., and David Cohen. "The Ethics of Electroconvulsive Therapy." *Ethics Journal of the American Medical Association* 5, no. 10 (2003).

Mowbray, R. M. "Historical Aspects of Electric Convulsant Therapy." *Scottish Medical Journal* 4 (1959): 373–378.

Mulsant, Benoit H., Roger F. Haskett, Joan Prudic, Michael E. Thase, Kevin M. Malone, J. John Mann, Helen M. Pettinati, and Harold A. Sackeim. "Low Use of Neuroleptic Drugs in the Treatment of Psychotic Major Depression." *American Journal of Psychiatry* 154, no. 4 (1997): 559–561.

Myerson, Abraham. "Borderline Cases Treated by Electric Shock." *American Journal of Psychiatry* 100 (1943): 355–357.

Nasar, Sylvia. *A Beautiful Mind: The Life of Mathematical Genius and Nobel Laureate John Nash.* New York: Simon & Schuster, 1994.

National Institutes of Health. "Electroconvulsive Therapy: National Institutes of Health Consensus Development Conference Statement." June 10–12, 1985, 5 (11): 1–23.

National Institutes of Health Consensus Development Panel on Depression in Late Life. "Diagnosis and Treatment of Depression in Late Life." *Journal of the American Medical Association* 268, no. 8 (August 26, 1992): 1018–1024.

Neylan, Thomas C., Jonathan D. Canick, Stephen E. Hall, Victor I. Reus, Robert M. Sapolsky, and Owen M. Wolkowitz. "Cortisol Levels Predict Cognitive Impairment Induced by Electroconvulsive Therapy." *Society of Biological Psychiatry* 50, no. 5 (September 2001): 331–336.

Nobler, Mitchell S., Maria A. Oquendo, Lawrence S. Kegeles, Kevin M. Malone, Carl Campbell, Harold A. Sackeim, and J. John Mann. "Decreased Regional

Brain Metabolism After ECT." *American Journal of Psychiatry* 158, no. 2 (2001): 305–308.

Nobler, Mitchell S., Charlotte C. Teneback, Ziad Nahas, Daryl E. Bohning, Ananda Shastri, F. Andrew Kozel, and Mark S. George. "Structural and Functional Neuroimaging of Electroconvulsive Therapy and Transcranial Magnetic Stimulation." *Depression and Anxiety* 12, no. 3 (2000): 144–156.

Norton, Paul. "Electroshock Stirs up Furor." *Capital Times,* November 3, 1995.

"Notes on Science: Stammering Cured by Electric Shock." *New York Times,* February 29, 1948, sec. E, p. 11.

Noyes, Arthur P. "Philadelphia Psychiatric Society, regular meeting Nov. 13, 1942." *Archives of Neurology and Psychiatry* 49 (1943): 786–791.

Nuland, Sherwin. *Lost in America: A Journey with My Father.* New York: Alfred A. Knopf, 2003.

———. E-mail to author, May 23, 2005.

Null, Gary. "An Overview of the Problem of Electroconvulsive Therapy." New York State Assembly Mental Health Committee. New York City, May 18, 2001.

Nuttall, Gregory A., Monique R. Bowersox, Stephanie B. Douglass, Jenny McDonald, Laura J. Rasmussen, Paul A. Decker, William C. Oliver, and Keith G. Rasmussen. "Morbidity and Mortality in the Use of Electroconvulsive Therapy." *Journal of ECT* 20, no. 4 (2004): 237–241.

O'Leary, Dennis A., and Alan S. Lee. "Seven-Year Prognosis in Depression Mortality and Readmission Risk in the Nottingham ECT Cohort." *British Journal of Psychiatry* 169, no. 4 (1996): 423–429.

O'Shea, Brian, and Aidan McGennis. "ECT: Lay Attitudes and Experiences—A Pilot Study." *Irish Medical Journal* 76, no. 1 (1983): 40–43.

Odejide, A. O., J. U. Ohaeri, and B. A. Ikuesan. "Electroconvulsive Therapy in Nigeria." *Convulsive Therapy* 3, no. 1 (1987): 31–37.

Ohaeri, Jude U., Cletus C. Hedo, Solomon N. Enyidah, and Adesola O. Ogunniyi. "Tissue Injury—Inducing Potential of Unmodified ECT: Serial Measurement of Acute Phase Reactants." *Convulsive Therapy* 8, no. 4 (1992): 253–257.

Olfson, Mark, Steven Marcus, Harold A. Sackeim, James Thompson, and Harold Alan Pincus. "Use of ECT for the Inpatient Treatment of Recurrent Major Depression." *American Journal of Psychiatry* 155, no. 1 (1998): 22–29.

One Flew Over the Cuckoo's Nest. Film. Directed by Milos Forman. Fantasy Films, 1975.

Ontario Health Technology Advisory Committee. "Repetitive Transcranial Magnetic Stimulation," June 17, 2004. Available at http://www.health.gov.on.ca/english/providers/program/mas/reviews/docs/recommend_rtms_061704.pdf.

Oquendo, Maria A., Masoud Kamali, Steven P. Ellis, Michael F. Grunebaum, Kevin M. Malone, Beth S. Brodsky, Harold A. Sackeim, and J. John Mann. "Adequacy of Antidepressant Treatment After Discharge and the Occurrence of Suicidal Acts in Major Depression: A Prospective Study." *American Journal of Psychiatry* 159, no. 10 (2002): 1746–1751.

Ottosson, Jan-Otto. "Is ECT an Ethical Treatment?" *Psychiatric Times,* March 1, 2004.

———. "Psychological or Physiological Theories of ECT." *International Journal of Psychiatry* 5, no. 2 (1968): 170–174.

Ottosson, Jan-Otto, and Max Fink. "A Dilemma in Ethics," Draft, October 24, 2003.

Pain, Stephanie. "Lady Emma's Shocking Past." *New Scientist,* May 10, 2003.

Palmer, Robert L., ed. *Electroconvulsive Therapy: An Appraisal.* New York: Oxford University Press, 1981.

Papolos, Demitri F., and Janice Papolos. *Overcoming Depression.* New York: Harper & Row, 1987.

Parmar, Ranjana. "Attitudes of Child Psychiatrists to Electroconvulsive Therapy." *Psychiatric Bulletin* 17 (1993): 12–13.

Parry, John. "Legal Parameters of Informed Consent Applied to Electroconvulsive Therapy." *Mental and Physical Disability Law Reporter* 9, no. 3. Available at http://www.ect.org/resources/summary.html.

Passione, Roberta. "Italian Psychiatry in an International Context: Ugo Cerletti and the Case of Electroshock." *History of Psychiatry* 15, no. 1 (2004): 83–104.

Paul, K-Lynn. "Electroshock." *Washington Post,* February 4, 1973, P08.

Peck, Robert E. *The Miracle of Shock Treatment.* Jericho, N.Y.: Exposition Press, 1974.

Pedler, Margaret., "Shock Treatment: A Survey of People's Experiences of Electro-Convulsive Therapy." *Mind: The Mental Health Charity.* March 2001.

Perry, Michael. "Horror Tales Emerge from Australian Hospital." *Jakarta Post,* December 28, 1990.

Pettinati, Helen M., Stephani M. Stephens, Kenneth M. Willis, and Sarah E. Robin. "Evidence for Less Improvement in Depression in Patients Taking Benzodiazepines During Unilateral ECT." *American Journal of Psychiatry* 147, no. 8 (August 1990): 1029–1035.

Philibert, Robert A., Larry Richards, Charles F. Lynch, and George Winokur. "Effect of ECT on Mortality and Clinical Outcome in Geriatric Unipolar Depression." *Journal of Clinical Psychiatry* 56, no. 9 (1995): 390–394.

Philpot, M., A. Treloar, N. Gormley, and L. Gustafson. "Barriers to the Use of Electroconvulsive Therapy in the Elderly: A European Survey." *European Psychiatry* 17, no. 1 (March 2002): 41–45.

Piersall, Jim, and Al Hirshberg. *Fear Strikes Out: The Jim Piersall Story.* Lincoln, Neb.: Bison Books, 1999.

Pippard, John. "Audit of Electroconvulsive Treatment in Two National Health Service Regions." *British of Psychiatry* 160 (1992): 621–637.

———. "ECT Custom and Practice." *Psychiatric Bulletin* 12, no. 11 (1988): 473–475.

Pirsig, Robert M. *Zen and the Art of Motorcycle Maintenance: An Inquiry into Values.* New York: William Morrow & Company, 1974.

Plath, Sylvia. *The Bell Jar.* London: Heinemann, 1963.

Polk, Hugh L. "Shock Therapy Still Causes Brain Damage." *New York Times,* August 1, 1993, sec. 4, p. 14.

Potter, William Z., and Matthew V. Rudorfer. "Electroconvulsive Therapy: A Modern Medical Procedure." Editorial. *New England Journal of Medicine* 328 (March 25, 1993): 882–883.

Pridmore, Saxby. "Substitution of Rapid Transcranial Magnetic Stimulation Treatments for Electroconvulsive Therapy Treatments in a Course of Electroconvulsive Therapy." *Depression and Anxiety* 12, no. 3 (2000): 118–123.

Prudic, Joan, Linda Fitzsimons, Mitchell S. Nobler, and Harold A. Sackeim. "Naloxone in the Prevention of the Adverse Cognitive Effects of ECT: A Within-Subject, Placebo Controlled Study." *Neuropsychopharmacology* 21, no. 2 (1999): 285–293.

Prudic, Joan, Roger Haskett, Benoit Mulsant, Kevin M. Malone, Helen Pettinati, Stephani Stephens, Robert Greenberg, Sheryl L. Rifas, and Harold A. Sackeim. "Resistance to Antidepressant Medications and Short-Term Clinical Response to ECT." *American Journal of Psychiatry* 153, no. 8 (1996): 985–992.

Prudic, Joan, Mark Olfson, Steven C. Marcus, Rice B. Fuller, and Harold A. Sackeim. "Effectiveness of Electroconvulsive Therapy in Community Settings." *Biological Psychiatry* 55, no. 2 (2004): 301–312.

Prudic, Joan, Mark Olfson, and Harold A. Sackeim. "Electro-Convulsive Therapy Practices in the Community." *Psychological Medicine* 31, no. 5 (2001): 929–934.

Prudic, Joan, Shoshana Peyser, and Harold A. Sackeim. "Subjective Memory Complaints: A Review of Patient Self-Assessment of Memory After Electroconvulsive Therapy." *Journal of ECT* 16, no. 2 (2000): 121–132.

Prudic, Joan, and Harold A. Sackeim. "Electroconvulsive Therapy and Suicide Risk." *Journal of Clinical Psychiatry* 60, supp. 2 (1999): 104–110.

Prudic, Joan, Harold A. Sackeim, and D. P. Devanand. "Medication Resistance and Clinical Response to Electroconvulsive Therapy." *Psychiatry Research* 31 (March 1990): 287–296.

Psychoanalytic Institute for Social Research, Rome, Italy. "Ethical Aspects of Coercive Supervision and/or Treatment of Uncooperative Psychiatric Patients in the Community, Italian Report," 1994.

Pulver, Sidney E. "The First Electroconvulsive Treatment Given in the United States." *American Journal of Psychiatry* 117 (March 1961): 845–846.

Rabin, Albert. "Patients Who Received More than One Hundred Electric Shock Treatments." *Journal of Personality* 17 (1948): 42–47.

Raj, Y. Pritham. "Medicine, Myths, and the Movies." *Post Graduate Medicine* 113, no. 6 (June 2003): 9–10, 13.

Ranganath, Rattehalli Dattatreya, Jagadisha, Bangalore Nanjudappa Gangadhar, Manish Tomar, Vittal Srinivas Candade, and Koodakanti Raghavaiah Hemalatha. "ECT and Heart Rate Changes: An Alternative to EEG Monitoring for Seizure Confirmation During Modified ECT." *German Journal of Psychiatry* 6, no. 3 (2003).

Raskin, David. "A Survey of Electroconvulsive Therapy: Use and Training in University Hospitals in 1984 (letter to editor)." *Convulsive Therapy* 2, no. 4 (1986): 293–299.

Rasmussen, Keith G., Shirlene M. Sampson, and Teresa A. Rummans. "Electroconvulsive Therapy and Newer Modalities for the Treatment of Medication-Refractory Mental Illness." *Mayo Clinic Proceedings* 77, no. 6 (2002): 552–556.

Read, John. "Electroconvulsive Therapy." In *Models of Madness: Psychological, Social and Biological Approaches to Schizophrenia.* Edited by John Read, Loren R. Mosher, and Richard P. Bentall, New York: Routledge, 2004.

Reid, William H., Sandy Keller, Martha Leatherman, and Mark Mason. "ECT in Texas: 19 Months of Mandatory Reporting." *Journal of Clinical Psychiatry* 59, no. 1 (1998): 8–13.

Relton, H. Louise. "Electroconvulsive Therapy: Patients Must be Confident that Evidence of Efficacy Is Compelling." *British Medical Journal* 327 (September 13, 2003): 621.

Remnick, David. "25 Years of Nightmares: Victims of CIA-Funded Mini Experiments Seek Damages from the Agency." *Washington Post,* July 28, 1985, sec. F1, p. 2.

Rey, Joseph M., and Garry Walter. "Half a Century of ECT Use in Young People." *American Journal of Psychiatry* 154, no. 5 (May 1997): 595–602.

Reynolds, Wellington, W. "Electric Shock Treatment: Observations in 350 Cases." *Psychiatric Quarterly* 19 (1945): 322–333.

Rice, Marilyn. "The Industry Wins." Letter to the Editor, *New York Times,* November 10, 1982.

Rose, Diana, Pete Fleischmann, Til Wykes, Morven Leese, and Jonathan Bindman. "Patients' Perspectives on Electroconvulsive Therapy: Systematic Review." *British Medical Journal* 326 (June 21, 2003): 1363.

Rose, Diana S., Til H. Wykes, Jonathan P. Bindman, and Pete S. Fleischmann. "Information, Consent and Perceived Coercion: Patients' Perspectives on Electroconvulsive Therapy." *British Journal of Psychiatry* 186 (2005): 54–59.

Rose, Diana, Til H. Wykes, Morven Leese, Jonathan Bindman, and Pete Fleischmann. "Patients' Perspectives on Electroconvulsive Therapy: Systematic Review." *British Medical Journal* 326 (June 21, 2003): 1363–1367.

Rosenbach, Margo L. Richard C. Hermann, and Robert A. Dorwart. "Use of Electroconvulsive Therapy in the Medicare Population Between 1987 and 1992." *Psychiatric Services* 48, no. 12 (December 1997): 1537–1542.

Rosenblatt, Jack E. "Interview with Max Fink." *Currents,* December 1993.

Rothschild, David, D. J. Van Gordon, and Anthony Varjabedian. "Regressive Shock Therapy in Schizophrenia." *Diseases of the Nervous System* 12, no. 5 (May 1951): 147–150.

"Royal College of Psychiatrists' Memorandum on the Use of Electroconvulsive Therapy, The." *British Journal of Psychiatry* 131 (1977): 261–268.

Roy-Byrne, Peter, and Robert H. Gerner. "Legal Restrictions on the Use of ECT in California: Clinical Impact on the Incompetent Patient." *Journal of Clinical Psychiatry* 42, no. 8 (1981): 300–303.

Rubenstein, Leonard S. "The C.I.A. and the Evil Doctor." *New York Times,* November 7, 1988, A-19.

Rudorfer, Matthew V. "Overview." *Psychopharmacology Bulletin* 30, no. 3 (1994): 261–264.

Rudorfer, Matthew V., Michael E. Henry, and Harold A. Sackeim. "Electroconvulsive Therapy." In *Psychiatry,* 2nd ed. Edited by Allan Tasman, Jerald Kay, and Jeffrey A. Lieberman. Hoboken, N.J.: John Wiley & Sons, 2003.

Rudorfer, Matthew V., and Barry D. Lebowitz. "Progress in ECT Research." *American Journal of Psychiatry* 156, no. 6 (June 1999): 975.

Rudorfer, Matthew V., Husseini K. Manji, and William Z. Potter. "ECT and Delirium in Parkinson's Disease." *American Journal of Psychiatry* 149, no. 12 (1992): 1758–1759.

Rudorfer, Matthew V., Emile D. Risby, John K. Hsiao, et al. "Disparate Biochemical Actions of Electroconvulsive Therapy and Antidepressant Drugs." *Convulsive Therapy* 4, no. 2 (1988): 133–140.

Ruffin, William C., J. T. Monroe, and Gordon E. Rader. "Attitudes of Auxiliary Personnel Administering Electroconvulsive and Insulin Coma Treatment: A Comparative Study." *Journal of Nervous and Mental Disease* 131 (1960): 241–246.

Rule, Sheila. "Looking Back at 1956: Passion, and Then Pain." *New York Times,* June 17, 1989, sec. 1, p. 6.

Rush, A. John, Mark S. George, Harold A. Sackeim, Lauren B. Marangell, Mustafa M. Husain, Cole Giller, Ziad Nahas, Stephen Haines, Richard K. Simpson Jr., and

Robert Goodman. "Vagus Nerve Stimulation (VNS) for Treatment-Resistant Depressions: A Multicenter Study." *Biological Psychiatry* 47, no. 4 (2000): 276–286.

Sackeim, Harold A. "Are ECT Devices Underpowered?" *Convulsive Therapy* 7, no. 4 (1991): 233–236.

———. "The Case for ECT." *Psychology Today* 19, no. 6 (June 1985): 37–40.

———. "Convulsant and Anticonvulsant Properties of Electroconvulsive Therapy: Toward a Focal Form of Brain Stimulation." *Clinical Neuroscience Research* 4 (2004): 39–57.

———. "Electroconvulsive Therapy: A New Age?" *Treatment Today* (Summer 1995): 39.

———. "Memory and ECT: From Polarization to Reconciliation." *Journal of ECT* 16, no. 2 (2000): 87–96.

Sackeim, Harold A., Paolo Decina, Maureen Kanzler, Barbara Kerr, and Sidney Malitz. "Effects of Electrode Placement on the Efficacy of Titrated, Low-Dose ECT." *American Journal of Psychiatry* 144, no. 11 (1987): 1449–1455.

Sackeim, Harold A., D. P. Devanand, and Joan Prudic. "Stimulus Intensity, Seizure Threshold, and Seizure Duration: Impact on the Efficacy and Safety of Electroconvulsive Therapy." *Psychiatric Clinics of North America* 14, no. 4 (1991): 803–843.

Sackeim, Harold A., Roger F. Haskett, Benoit H. Mulsant, Mitchell E. Thase, J. John Mann, Helen M. Pettinati, Robert M. Greenberg, Raymond R. Crowe, Thomas B. Cooper, and Joan Prudic. "Continuation Pharmacotherapy in the Prevention of Relapse Following Electroconvulsive Therapy: A Randomized Control Trial." *Journal of the American Medical Association* 285, no. 10 (2001): 1299–1307.

Sackeim, Harold A., Joan Prudic, D. P. Devanand, Mitchel S. Nobler, Sarah H. Lisanby, Shoshana Peyser, Linda Fitzsimons, Bobba J. Moody, and Jenifer Clark. "A Prospective, Randomized, Double-Blind Comparison of Bilateral and Right Unilateral Electroconvulsive Therapy at Different Stimulus Intensities." *Archives of General Psychiatry* 57, no. 5 (2000): 425–434.

Sackeim, Harold A., Joan Prudic, D. P. Devanand, Paolo Decina, Barbara Kerr, and Sidney Malitz. "The Impact of Medication Resistance and Continuation Pharmacology on Relapse Following Response to Electroconvulsive Therapy in Major Depression." *Journal of Clinical Psychopharmacology* 10, no. 2 (1990): 96–104.

Sackeim, Harold A., Joan Prudic, D. P. Devanand, Judith E. Kiersky, Linda Fitzsimons, Bobba J. Moody, Martin C. McElhiney, Eliza A. Coleman, and Joy M. Settembrino. "Effects of Stimulus Intensity and Electrode Placement on the Efficacy and Cognitive Effects of Electroconvulsive Therapy." *New England Journal of Medicine* 328 (March 25, 1993): 839–846.

Sackeim, Harold A., Joan Prudic, Rice Fuller, John Keilp, Philip W. Lavori, and Mark

Olfson. "The Cognitive Effects of Electroconvulsive Therapy in Community Settings." [Awaiting publication.]

Sackeim, Harold A., A. John Rush, Mark S. George, Lauren B. Marangell, Mustafa M. Husain, Ziad Nahas, Christopher R. Johnson, Stuart Seidman, Cole Giller, Stephen Haines, Richard K. Simpson Jr., and Robert R. Goodman. "Vagus Nerve Stimulation (VNS) for Treatment-Resistant Depression: Efficacy, Side Effects, and Predictors of Outcome." *Neuropsychopharmacology* 25, no. 5 (2001): 713–728.

Salford Community Health Council. *Electro-Convulsive Therapy: Its Use and Effects.* Manchester, UK: Salford Community Health Council, 1998. Available at http://www.healthyplace.com/Communities/Depression/ect/resources/UKreport.asp.

Salzman, Carl. "ECT and Ethical Psychiatry." *American Journal of Psychiatry* 134, no. 10 (September 1977): 1006–1009.

———. "ECT, Research, and Professional Ambivalence." *American Journal of Psychiatry* 155, no. 1 (January 1998): 1–2.

Salzman, Leon. "An Evaluation of Shock Therapy." *American Journal of Psychiatry* 103 (1947): 669–679.

Satcher, David. *Mental Health: A Report of the Surgeon General.* Washington, D.C.: U.S. Department of Health and Human Services, 1999.

Schmeck Jr., Harold M. "Memory Loss Linked to Electroshocks." *New York Times,* November 10, 1973, p. 6.

Scott, Allan I. F., Morag Gardner, and Rena Good. "Fall in ECT Use in Young People in Edinburgh." *Journal of ECT* 21, no. 1 (2005): 50.

Scott, Allan I. F., Colin R. Rodger, Ruth H. Stocks, and Anne P. Shering. "Is Old-Fashioned Electroconvulsive Therapy More Efficacious? A Randomised Comparative Study of Bilateral Brief-Pulse and Bilateral Sine-Wave Treatments." *British Journal of Psychiatry* 160 (1992): 360–364.

Selby Jr., Hubert. *Requiem for a Dream.* New York: Thunder's Mouth Press, 2000.

Selinski, Herman. "The Selective Use of Electro-shock Therapy as an Adjuvant to Psychotherapy." *Bulletin of the New York Academy of Medicine* (April 1943): 245–251.

Shapira, Baruch, Nurith Tubi, Heinz Drexler, David Lidsky, Avraham Calev, and Bernard Lerer. "Cost and Benefit in the Choice of ECT Schedule: Twice Versus Three Times Weekly ECT." *British Journal of Psychiatry* 172, no. 1 (1998): 44–48.

Sharma, Verinder. "Retrospective Controlled Study of Inpatient ECT: Does It Prevent Suicide?" *Journal of Affective Disorders* 56, nos. 2–3 (1999): 183–187.

Sharp, Lewis I., Anthony R. Gabriel, and David J. Impastato. "Management of the Acutely Disturbed Patient by Sedative Electroshock Therapy." *Diseases of the Nervous System* 14, no. 1 (1953): 21–24.

Shiwach, Raj S., William H. Reid, and Thomas J. Carmody. "An Analysis of Reported Deaths Following Electroconvulsive Therapy in Texas, 1993–1998." *Psychiatric Services* 52, no. 8 (2001): 1095–1097.

Shock Corridor. Film. Written, directed, and produced by Samuel Fuller. Criterion, 1963.

"Shock Treatment Cures Infidelity: Briton Loses Infatuation for a Neighbor's Wife." *New York Times,* December 4, 1966.

Shorter, Edward. "The History of ECT: Some Unsolved Mysteries." *Psychiatric Times* 21, no. 2 (February 2004).

———. *A History of Psychiatry: From the Era of the Asylum to the Age of Prozac.* New York: John Wiley & Sons, 1997.

Simini, Bruno. "Electroconvulsive Therapy Is Restricted in Italy." *Lancet* 353 (March 20, 1999): 993.

Simon, Robert I. "A Clinician's Perspective." *Psychiatric Times,* January 1, 2004, p. 45.

Skrabanek, Petr. "Convulsive Therapy—A Critical Appraisal of Its Origins and Value." *Irish Medical Journal* 79, no 6 (1986): 156–165.

Small, J. G., M. H. Klapper, J. J. Kellams, M. J. Miller, V. Milstein, P. H. Sharpley, and I. F. Small. "Electroconvulsive Treatment Compared with Lithium in the Management of Manic States." *Archives of General Psychiatry* 45, no. 8 (August 1988): 727–732.

Smith, Craig S. "Abuse of Electroshock Found in Turkish Mental Hospitals." *New York Times,* national edition, September 29, 2005, p. 3.

Smith, Daniel. "Shock and Disbelief." *The Atlantic Monthly,* February 1, 2001, p. 79.

Smith, Mark. "Profitable Addictions: Nightmare from '60s Haunts Mental Patients of '90s." *Houston Chronicle,* March 8, 1992, sec. A, p. 1.

Smith, Stephen. "Shock Therapy Aiding Kitty Dukakis." *Boston Globe,* July 24, 2003, B1.

Snake Pit, The. Film. Directed by Anatole Litvak. Twentieth Century Fox, 1948.

Sobin, Christina, Joan Prudic, D. P. Devanand, Mitchell S. Nobler, and Harold A. Sackeim. "Who Responds to ECT?: A Comparison of Effective and Ineffective Forms of Treatment." *British Journal of Psychiatry* 169, no. 3 (September 1996): 322–328.

Sobin, Christina, Harold A. Sackeim, Joan Prudic, D. P. Devanand, Bobba J. Moody, and Martin C. McElhiney. "Predictors of Retrograde Amnesia Following ECT." *American Journal of Psychiatry* 152, no. 7 (1995): 995–1001.

Squire, Larry R. "Memory Function as Affected by Electroconvulsive Therapy." *Annals of New York Academy of Science* 462 (1986): 307–314.

Squire, Larry R., and Pamela C. Slater. "Electroconvulsive Therapy and Complaints of Memory Dysfunction: A Prospective Three-Year Follow-up Study." *British Journal of Psychiatry* 142 (1983): 1–8.

"States' Rights vs. Victims' Rights." *New York Times,* May 8, 1977, p. 146.

Staudt, Virginia M., and Joseph Zubin. "A Biometric Evaluation of the Somatotherapies in Schizophrenia." *Psychological Bulletin* 54, no. 3 (1957): 171–196.

Sterling, Peter. "ECT Damage Is Easy to Find If You Look for It." *Nature* 403, no. 6767 (2000): 242.

Stern, Robert A., Charles T. Nevels, Mark E. Shelhorse, Mark L. Prohaska, George A. Mason, and Arthur J. Prang Jr.. "Antidepressant and Memory Effects of Combined Thyroid Hormone Treatment and Electroconvulsive Therapy: Preliminary Findings." *Biological Psychiatry* 30, no. 6 (1991): 623–627.

Stevens, Lawrence. "Psychiatry's Electroconvulsive SHOCK TREATMENT: A Crime Against Humanity." Available at http://www.antipsychiatry.org.

Strain, J. J., L. Brunschwig, J. P. Duffy, D. P. Agle, A. L. Rosenbaum, and T. G. Ridder. "Comparison of Therapeutic Effects and Memory Changes with Bilateral and Unilateral ECT." *American Journal of Psychiatry* 125, no. 3 (1968): 50–60.

Strober, Michael, Uma Rao, Mark DeAntonio, Edward Liston, Matthew State, Lisa Amaya-Jackson, and Sara Latz. "Effects of Electroconvulsive Therapy in Adolescents with Severe Endogenous Depression Resistant to Pharmacotherapy." *Biological Psychiatry* 43, no. 5 (1998): 335–338.

Stromgren, L. S. "Electroconvulsive Therapy in the Nordic Countries, 1977–1987." *Acta Psychiatrica Scandinavica* 84, no. 5 (November 1991): 428–434.

Styron, William. *Darkness Visible: A Memoir of Madness.* New York: Random House, 1990.

Substance Abuse and Mental Health Services Administration. "Electroconvulsive Therapy Background Paper." Washington, D.C.: Department of Health and Human Services, March 1998.

Superior Court of the State of California for the County of Santa Barbara, Case No. 1069713, *Atze Akkerman and Elizabeth Akkerman vs Joseph Johnson,* Santa Barbara Cottage Hospital, et al., January 2, 2005, decision.

Szasz, Thomas S. *The Myth of Mental Illness: Foundations of a Theory of Personal Conduct.* New York: Harper & Row, 1974.

Szuba, Martin P., Lewis R. Baxter, Edward H. Liston, and Peter Roy-Byrne. "Patient and Family Perspectives of Electroconvulsive Therapy: Correlation with Outcome." *Convulsive Therapy* 7, no. 3 (1991): 175–183.

Taieb, Olivier, David Cohen, Philippe Mazet, and Martine Flament. "Adolescents' Experiences with ECT." *Journal of the American Academy of Child and Adolescent Psychiatry* 39, no. 8 (2000): 943–944.

Taieb, Olivier, Martine F. Flament, Maurice Corcos, Philippe Jeammet, Michel Basquin, Philippe Mazet, and David Cohen. "Electroconvulsive Therapy in Adolescents with Mood Disorder: Patients' and Parents' Attitudes." *Psychiatry Research* 104, no. 2 (2001): 183–190.

Tannery, Bryan L. "Electroconvulsive Therapy and Suicide." *Suicide & Life-Threatening Behavior* 16, no. 2 (Summer 1986): 116–140.

Teles, A., and R. Benadhira. "Current Status of Electroconvulsive Therapy in Adult Psychiatric Care in France." *Encephale* 27, no. 2 (March/April 2001): 129–136.

Templer, Donald I., and David M. Veleber. "Can ECT Permanently Harm the Brain?" *Clinical Neuropsychology* 4, no. 2 (1982): 62–66.

Tew, James D., Benoit H. Mulsant, Roger F. Haskett, Joan Prudic, Michael E. Thase, Raymond R. Crowe, Diana Dolata, Amy E. Begley, Charles F. Reynolds, and Harold A. Sackeim. "Acute Efficacy of ECT in the Treatment of Major Depression in the Old-Old." *American Journal of Psychiatry* 156, no. 12 (December 1999): 1865–1870.

Texas Department of Mental Health and Mental Retardation, "Annual Report on Electroconvulsive Therapy in Texas," fiscal years 1994–2004.

Thomas, Gordon. *Journey into Madness: Medical Torture and the Mind Controllers.* London: Corgi Books, 1988.

Thompson, James W., and Jack D. Blaine. "Use of ECT in the United States in 1975 and 1980." *American Journal of Psychiatry* 144 (May 1987): 557–562.

Thompson, James W., Richard D. Weiner, and C. Patrick Myers. "Use of ECT in the United States in 1975, 1980, and 1986." *American Journal of Psychiatry* 151 (November 1994): 1657–1661.

Thomson-Medstat. "MarketScan Commercial Claims and Encounters and Medicare Supplemental Databases 1991, 1996, 2001, 2003: Counts of Patients with Electroconvulsive Therapy." Data analysis run for authors, Cambridge, Massachusetts, 2005.

Tierney, Gene, and Mickey Herskowitz. *Self-Portrait.* New York: Wyden Books, 1979.

Tillotson, Kenneth J., and Wolfgang Sulzbach. "A Comparative Study and Evaluation of Electric Shock Therapy in Depressive States." *American Journal of Psychiatry* 101, no. 4 (January 1945): 455–459.

Triebwasser, Joseph, and Richard Hersh. "Cost-effective." *New York Times,* August 1, 1993.

Trivedi, Madhukar H., A. John Rush, Stephen R. Wisniewski, Andrew A. Nierenberg, Diane Warden, Louise Ritz, Grayson Norquist, Robert H. Howland, Barry Lebowitz, Patrick J. McGrath, Kathy Shores-Wilson, Melanie M. Biggs, G. K. Balasubramani, and Maurizio Fava. "Evaluation of Outcomes with Citalopram for Depression Using Measurement-Based Care in STAR*D: Implications for Clinical Practice," *American Journal of Psychiatry* 163:1 (January 2006): 1–13.

"Truth in Psychiatry: Electroconvulsive Study Challenged." *Mental Health Law Weekly,* December 11, 2004.

UK ECT Review Group. "Efficacy and Safety of Electroconvulsive Therapy in Depressive Disorders: A Systematic Review and Meta-Analysis." *Lancet* 361 (March 8, 2003): 799–808.

Unger, Roger. "Shock Therapy Unsafe, Inhumane." *Register-Guard* (Eugene, Oregon), April 5, 1995, p. 11A.

U.S. Food and Drug Administration, Docket 1982P-0316, 1984P-0430, ECT files.

———. Letter from FDA Commissioner Donald Kennedy to Peter Sterling at the University of Pennsylvania, February 15, 1979, Public Document Room, File 78N-1103.

Vallance, M. "The Experience of Electro-Convulsive Therapy by a Practising Psychiatrist." *British Journal of Psychiatry* 111 (April 1965): 365–367.

Van Atta, Winfred. *Shock Treatment.* New York: Doubleday, 1961.

Van de Water, Marjorie. "Electric Shock, a New Treatment." *Science News Letter* (July 20, 1940): 42–44.

van der Wurff, F. B., M. L. Stek, W.J.G. Hoogendijk, and A.T.F. Beekman. "The Efficacy and Safety of ECT in Depressed Older Adults, a Literature Review." *International Journal of Geriatric Psychiatry* 18 (2003): 894–904.

van Waarde, Jeroen A., Joost J. Stolker, and Rose C. van der Mast. "ECT in Mental Retardation: A Review." *Journal of ECT* 17, no. 4 (2001): 236–243.

Vermont Department of Developmental and Mental Health Services. "Informed Consent Package for Electroconvulsive Therapy." Montpelier, Vt.: revised 10/2001 and 11/2004.

Vermont Department of Health, Division of Mental Health. "Annual Data on Electroconvulsive Therapy," Fiscal Years 2001–2004.

Vest, David. "Remembering Tammy Wynette." *Birmingham News,* April 12, 1998.

Vieweg, Reinout, and Charles R. Shawcross. "A Trial to Determine Any Difference Between Two and Three Times a Week ECT in the Rate of Recovery from Depression." *Journal of Mental Health* 7, no. 4 (1998): 403–409.

Wai-Kwong Tang, and Gabor S. Ungvari. "Electroconvulsive Therapy in Rehabilitation: The Hong Kong Experience." *Psychiatric Services* 52 (March 2001): 303–306.

Walker, Ray, and Conrad Melton Swartz. "Electroconvulsive Therapy During High-Risk Pregnancy." *General Hospital Psychiatry* 16, no. 5 (1994): 348–353.

Wallcraft, J. "Women & ECT." *Spare Rib,* October 1987.

Walling, Anne D. "Is It Time to Reconsider Use of ECT for Depression? Tips from Other Journals." *American Family Physician* (November 15, 2003).

Walter, Garry, Karryn Koster, and Joseph M. Rey. "Electroconvulsive Therapy in Adolescents: Experience, Knowledge, and Attitudes of Recipients." *Journal of the American Academy of Child & Adolescent Psychiatry* 38, no. 5 (May 1999): 594–599.

———. "Views about Treatment among Parents of Adolescents Who Received Electroconvulsive Therapy." *Psychiatric Services* 50, no. 5 (1999): 701–702.

Walter, Garry, and Andrew McDonald. "About to Have ECT? Fine, but Don't Watch It in the Movies: The Sorry Portrayal of ECT in Film." *Psychiatric Times* 21, no. 7 (June 1, 2004).

Walter, Garry, and Joseph M. Rey. "An Epidemiological Study of the Use of ECT in Adolescents." *Journal of the American Academy of Child & Adolescent Psychiatry* 36, no. 6 (June 1997): 807–815.

Ward, Mary Jane. *The Snake Pit.* New York: Random House, 1946.

Warren, Carol A. B. "Electroconvulsive Therapy, the Self, and Family Relations." *Research in the Sociology of Health Care* 7 (1988): 283–300.

Wasserman, Dale. *One Flew Over the Cuckoo's Nest: A Play in Two Acts.* New York: Samuel French, Inc., 1970.

Wasserman, Eric M. "Side Effects of Repetitive Transcranial Magnetic Stimulation." *Depression and Anxiety* 12 (2000): 124–129.

Wasserman, Eric M., and Sarah H. Lisanby. "Therapeutic Application of Repetitive Transcranial Magnetic Stimulation: A Review." *Clinical Neurophysiology* 112, no. 8 (August 2001): 1367–1377.

Weiner, Richard D. "Does Electroconvulsive Therapy Cause Brain Damage?" *Behavioral and Brain Sciences* 7 (1984): 1–53.

Weiner, Richard D., and C. Edward Coffey. "Electroconvulsive Therapy in the United States." *Psychopharmacology Bulletin* 27, no. 1 (1991): 9–15.

Weiner, Richard D., Helen J. Rogers, Jonathan R. T. Davidson, and Larry R. Squire. "Effects of Stimulus Parameters on Cognitive Side Effects." *Annals of New York Academy of Science* 462 (1986): 315–325.

Weitz, Don. "Electroshocking Elderly People: Another Psychiatric Abuse." *Changes: An International Journal of Psychology and Psychotherapy* 15, no. 2 (May 1997).

Welch, Charles A. "Electroconvulsive Therapy in the General Hospital." In *Massachusetts General Hospital Handbook of General Hospital Psychiatry,* 5th ed. Edited by Theodore A. Stern. Cambridge, Ma.: Mosby, 2004.

Wertz, Elizabeth. "The Fury of Shock Treatment—a Patient's View." *Washington Post,* December 10, 1972, PO36, p. 5.

West, Eric D. "Electric Convulsion Therapy in Depression: A Double-Blind Controlled Trial." *British Medical Journal* 282, no. 6275 (1981): 355–357.

Westfield, John Cloud. "New Sparks over Electroshock." *Time,* February 26, 2001.

Westphal, James R., Ronald Horswell, Sanjaya Kumar, and Jill Rush. "Quantifying Utilization and Practice Variation of Electroconvulsive Therapy." *Convulsive Therapy* 13, no. 4 (1997): 242–252.

Whitaker, Robert. *Mad in America: Bad Science, Bad Medicine, and the Enduring Mistreatment of the Mentally Ill.* New York: Perseus Publishing, 2002.

"Who Knocks Shocks?" *Psychology Today.* November–December 1995.

Wilkinson, David, and Janet Daoud. "The Stigma and the Enigma of ECT." *International Journal of Geriatric Psychiatry* 13, no. 12 (1998): 833–855.

Will, Otto Allen, Frederick Cooper Rehfeldt, and Meta A. Neumann. "A Fatality in Electroshock Therapy: Report of a Case and Review of Certain Previously Described Cases." *Journal of Nervous and Mental Disease* 107 (1948): 105–126.

Williams, Justin H. G., John T. O'Brien, and Sarah Cullum. "Time Course of Response to Electroconvulsive Therapy in Elderly Depressed Subjects." *International Journal of Geriatric Psychiatry* 12, no. 5 (1977): 563–566.

Winslade, William J., Edward H. Liston, Judith Wilson Ross, and Katherine D. Weber. "Medical, Judicial, and Statutory Regulation of ECT in the United States." *American Journal of Psychiatry* 141, no. 11 (November 1984): 1349–1355.

Wise, Jacuqi. "ECT Clinics Are Below Standard." *British Medical Journal* 314 (January 25, 1997): 247.

Wood, Debra A., and Philip M. Burgess. "Epidemiological Analysis of ECT in Victoria, Australia." *Australian and New Zealand Journal of Psychiatry* 37, no. 3 (June 2003): 307–311.

Youssef, Hanafy. "The Death of Electroconvulsive Therapy." *Advances in Therapy* 18, no. 2 (2001): 83–89.

———. "Time to Abandon Electroconvulsion as a Treatment in Modern Psychiatry." *Advances in Therapy* 16, no. 1 (1999): 29–38.

Zamora, Emil N., and Rudolf Kaelbling. "Memory and Electroconvulsive Therapy." *American Journal of Psychiatry* 122 (November 1965): 546–554.

Zervas, Iannis M., and Max Fink. "ECT and Delirium in Parkinson's Disease." *American Journal of Psychiatry* 149, no. 12 (1992): 1758.

Zimmerman, Mark, William Coryell, Bruce Pfohl, Caryn Corenthal, and Dalene Stangl. "ECT Response in Depressed Patients with and without a DSM-III Personality Disorder." *American Journal of Psychiatry* 143, no. 8 (1986): 1030–1032.

Author E-mails

Dr. Richard Abrams, Dr. Chittaranjan Andrade, Linda Andre, Sister Barbara, Dr. Kerry Bloomingdale, Dr. Tom Bolwig, Ted Chabasinski, Heather Cobb, Barbara Collins-Layton, Paul Cumming, Dr. Catherine Datto, Dr. Stephen Dinwiddie, Anne Donahue, Thomas Eagleton, Dr. Terry Early, Dr. Max Fink, Leonard Roy Frank, Dr. Sergio Grozavu, June Judge, Susan Kaplan, Dr. Charles Kellner, Nancy Kopans, Dr. Barry Alan Kramer, Peter Lehmann, Cindy Lepore, Dr. Benjamin Liptzin, Dr. Sarah Lisanby, William Marder, Dr. Robert Mayer, Dr. W. Vaughn McCall, Kathryn Cohan McNulty, Robin Nicol, Dr. Sherwin Nuland, David Oaks, Dr. Robert Palmer, Dr. Alvaro Pascual-Leone, Gloria Pope, Dr. Joan Prudic, Margo Rosenbach, Dr. Jerrold Rosenbaum, Dr. Leon Rosenberg, Dr. Harold Sackeim, Gail Schifsky, Dr. Steven Shon, Sara Stanfill, Joseph Stone, Deborah Thomas, Dr. Richard Weiner, Dr. Tony Weiner, and Dr. Charles Welch, Glenna Wheeler, Robert Whitaker, and Eileen White.

Author Interviews

ECT patients and family members: Kathy Bashor, Andy Behrman, Kim Billington, Ann Brennan, Sylvia Caras, Connie Clark, Sue Clark, Barbara Collins-Layton, Debbie Connolly, Paul Cumming, Sheri de Grom, Carrie DeLoach, Marie DeRose, Anne Donahue, Andrea Dukakis, John Dukakis, Kara Dukakis, Kitty Dukakis, Michael Dukakis, Christine Elvidge, Rhoda Falk, Lenny Ferguson, Dr. Judith Ferko, Louise Finocchio, Richard Finocchio, Joanne Fitzgerald, Thomas Fitzgerald, Lorraine Fougere, Raymond Fougere, James R. Giger, Rosemarie Goodwin, Frank Grant, Christina Heath, Mike Henry, Faye Johnson, Thomas Johnson, Karren S. Jones, June Judge, Susan Kadis, Kaj-Willow Kaemmerer, Steven A. Katz, Rich Kensinger, Joe Kerouac, Geraldine Knaack, Nancy Kopans, Shirley Lake, Pam Landry, Carmen Lee, Emily Lewis, Fred Lewis, Martha Manning, Ava Martinez, Andy Marx, Kathy Marx, Kathryn Cohan McNulty, Eileen Mowles, Donna Orrin, Marlene Paterson, Catherine Pemberton, Al Peters, Jinny Peters, Marc Pierre, Julia Prentice, Dr. Leon Rosenberg, Boyd Roth, Lucy Sajdak, Karen Schiller, Julaine Siegel, Leslie Sladek-Sobczak, Sara Stanfill, Cliff Steele, Catherine Steinhoff, Katie Steinhoff, Fred Stephens, Rose Styron, William Styron, Archie Walker, Bonita Walker-Jones, Marcy Walraven, Laurie Weist, Eileen White, Greg Wild, Shirley Willett, Alisson Wood, and Laurel Zangerl. Also Sister Barbara, Carolyn, Heidi, Jon, Steve L., Valerie, and many others who asked that neither their last nor first names be used.

   ECT doctors, critics, and others familiar with the procedure or with patients who received it: Dr. Musbau Abdulai, Dr. Howard Abrams, Dr. Danielle Anderson, Linda Andre,

Sandy Bakalar, Corky Balzac, Dr. Kerry Bloomingdale, Dr. Tom Bolwig, Dr. Jonathan Brodie, Ted Chabasinski, Dr. Beth Childs, Dr. Bruce Cohen, Paul Costello, Dr. Stephen Dinwiddie, Dr. Terry Early, Anne Fetherman, Dr. Max Fink, Dr. Herbert Fox, Leonard Roy Frank, Wilma Greenfield, Dr. Michael Henry, Dr. Richard Hermann, A. E. Hotchner, Dr. Sergio Grozavu, Dr. Keith Isenberg, Kay Redfield Jamison, Dr. Philip Janicak, Dr. Thomas Jewitt, Dr. Charles Kellner, Dr. Descartes Li, Dr. Benjamin Liptzin, Dr. Sarah Lisanby, Frederick Magnavito, Dr. John Matthews, Dr. W. Vaughn McCall, Maureen McGlame, David Mirkovich, Dr. Frank Moscarillo, Dr. Thomas Neylan, Robin Nicol, David Oaks, Dr. Larry Park, Dr. Alvaro Pascual-Leone, Al Peters, Jinny Peters, Dr. Judith Livant Rapoport, Margo Rosenbach, Dr. Matthew Rudorfer, Dr. Harold Sackeim, Dr. Alan Schatzberg, Dr. Stephen Seiner, Angelina Szot, Dr. Rajiv Tandon, Julie Totten, Dr. Richard Weiner, Dr. Tony Weiner, Dr. Roger Weiss, and Dr. Charles Welch.

INDEX